Renal Medicine

pocket tutor

JP

Renal Medicine

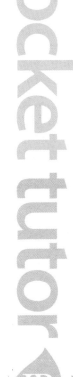

pocket tutor

David Oliveira PhD FRCP
Professor of Renal Medicine
St George's University of London
London, UK

Debasish Banerjee MD FRCP FASN
Consultant Nephrologist, Clinical Subdean
St George's Healthcare NHS Trust
Honorary Senior Lecturer
St George's University of London
London, UK

Joyce Popoola PhD MRCP
Consultant Nephrologist and Honorary Senior Lecturer
St George's Healthcare NHS Trust, London, UK

Iain A.M. MacPhee DPhil FRCP
Reader in Renal Medicine
Honorary Consultant Nephrologist
St George's University of London
London, UK

Seema Shrivastava PhD MRCP FHEA
Consultant Nephrologist and Honorary Senior Lecturer
St George's Healthcare NHS Trust
London, UK

Daniel Jones PhD FRCP
Consultant Nephrologist and Honorary Senior Lecturer
St George's Healthcare NHS Trust
London, UK

Stephen Nelson MD FRCP
Consultant Nephrologist, St George's Healthcare NHS Trust
London, UK

JP
medical
publishers

© 2013 JP Medical Ltd.

Published by JP Medical Ltd, 83 Victoria Street, London, SW1H 0HW, UK

Tel: +44 (0)20 3170 8910 Fax: +44 (0)20 3008 6180

Email: info@jpmedpub.com Web: www.jpmedpub.com

ISBN: 978-1-907816-57-4

British Library Cataloguing in Publication Data
A catalogue record for this book is available from the British Library

Library of Congress Cataloging in Publication Data
A catalog record for this book is available from the Library of Congress

JP Medical Ltd is a subsidiary of Jaypee Brothers Medical Publishers (P) Ltd, New Delhi, India.

Publisher:	Richard Furn
Development Editor:	Paul Mayhew
Design:	Designers Collective Ltd

Typeset, printed and bound in India.

Preface

Renal medicine is an area that tends to cause uncertainty, if not actual fear, in the minds of many undergraduates (and postgraduates, for that matter). It is true that areas such as glomerular disease, acid-base balance, and electrolyte disorders are complex, and the temptation is to leave them to the specialists. On the other hand, acute kidney injury is a common and often preventable occurrence amongst hospital inpatients, and the growing burden, both clinical and economic, of chronic kidney disease is an issue for primary and secondary care alike.

Despite the importance of renal medicine, we often struggle when asked by our students for suggestions for further reading. The standard general medical text books often do not, in our view, offer clear explanations of some of the more complex areas, and the large multi-volume texts are not really suitable for the non-specialist. With *Pocket Tutor Renal Medicine* we have attempted to fill the gap by providing information at the level that we would expect a final year student or newly qualified doctor to acquire. The book should also be suitable for other members of the multi-disciplinary team involved in the care of renal patients.

David Oliveira
Debasish Banerjee
Joyce Popoola
Iain A.M. MacPhee
Seema Shrivastava
Daniel Jones
Stephen Nelson
September 2012

Contents

First principles

The renal system and associated diseases are considered complex, even by many more senior doctors. This is probably due to the unique development and multiple functions of the urinary tract in comparison with other organ systems. An understanding of the first principles of the urinary tract, however, will make the understanding of the diseases and their management readily accessible to even the preclinical medical student.

1.1 Overview of the renal system

The urinary tract consists of two kidneys, two ureters and the single, centrally located bladder and urethra (**Figure 1.1**). Each kidney contains over a million **nephrons**, the functional units of the kidney. These are composed of glomeruli and tubules. The **tubules** join up as the renal collecting system to establish continuity with the rest of the renal tract. They are responsible for the physiological function of the renal tract, that is, regulation of the volume and composition of our body fluids. Tubules have several distinct epithelial cell types requiring precise positioning during fetal development in order to form an optimally functional urinary tract.

The urinary tract's main roles include excretion of waste products from the system (i.e. urine formation) and homeostasis of the extracellular environment by regulation of fluid balance and electrolyte concentration within the extracellular and intracellular compartments. The kidney is also responsible for the production of hormones such as erythropoietin, involved in the formation of red blood cells; the enzyme renin, a key player in blood pressure control and sodium reabsorption; and conversion of vitamin D to its active form dihydroxycholecalciferol, required for bone health.

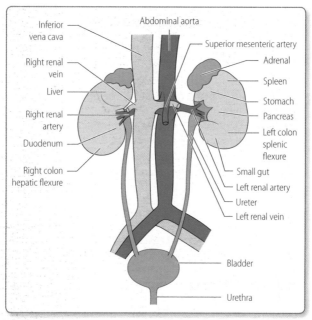

Figure 1.1 The urinary tract and its relations.

1.2 Anatomy and embryology

The kidneys

The kidneys are bean-shaped with concave **hila** (**Figures 1.2** and **1.3**). They are located retroperitoneally in the posterior abdominal wall at the level of T11 to L3 or L4 at either side of the lumbar vertebrae.

Relations

The relations of the kidney are:

- The diaphragm, quadratus lumborum, psoas, transversus abdominis, the 12th rib and the subcostal (T12), iliohypo-gastric and ilioinguinal nerves (L1) lie posteriorly

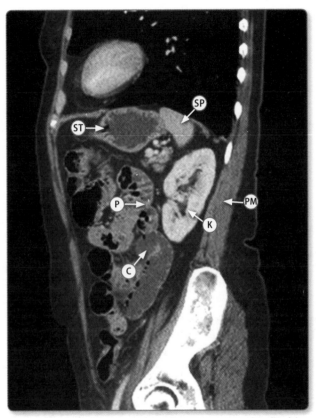

Figure 1.2 Sagittal computed tomography (CT) scan of the abdomen showing the left kidney and its relations. (**ST**) stomach, (**SP**) spleen, (**PM**) psoas muscle, (**P**) pancreas, (**C**) left colon, (**K**) left kidney.

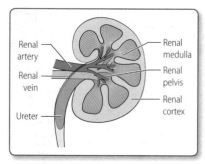

Figure 1.3 Gross anatomy and excretory function of the kidney. The renal artery brings in blood with excess water and toxins; blood leaves the kidney via the renal vein to the inferior vena cava. The removed excess water and toxins leave the kidney via the ureters to the bladder.

- The second part of the duodenum, ascending colon and the liver lie in front of the right kidney, while the left lies behind the stomach, pancreas, spleen and the descending colon
- Superiorly, both kidneys are closely capped by the adrenal glands
- The medial aspect of the hilum receives the **renal vein**, **renal artery** and **pelvis of the ureter** in that order as well as lymphatics and nerves

Clinical insight

In the past, most nephrectomies were carried out via an oblique incision midway between the 12th rib and iliac crest. Nowadays, they are increasingly done using minimally invasive laparoscopic surgery, especially in live kidney donors.

The surface anatomy of the kidneys is shown in **Figure 1.4**.

In adulthood, each normal kidney usually measures between 10 cm and 14 cm long and 6 cm wide depending on height and sex. The right kidney lies about 12 mm lower than the left, as it is displaced downwards by the liver. The kidneys are surrounded by perirenal fat, which has a protective role in supporting and cushioning the kidney.

Nerve supply

The nerve supply is particularly important in the kidney because it is essential for function in terms of regulation of vasomotor tone, which in turn regulates renal blood flow. The kidneys have a sympathetic supply arising from the lower splanchnic nerves,

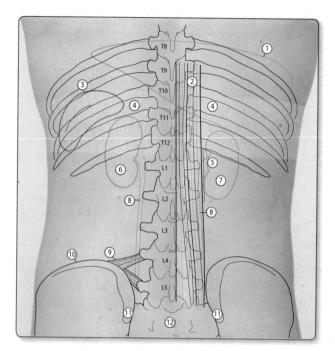

Figure 1.4 Surface anatomy and relations of the kidneys. ① Liver, ② erector spinae muscle group, ③ spleen, ④ region of costodiaphragmatic recess (white hatch), ⑤ renal angle, ⑥ left kidney, ⑦ right kidney, ⑧ ureter, ⑨ iliolumbar ligament, ⑩ iliac crest, ⑪ posterior superior iliac spine, ⑫ sacrum.

which travel through the lumbar ganglion to the kidney. Sympathetic stimulation leads to intrarenal vasoconstriction and hence reduced blood flow along side enhanced sodium reabsorption and stimulation of the local renin–angiotensin system.

Blood supply

The kidneys receive just over 20% of the cardiac output. Blood enters the kidney via the renal artery at the hilum. Renal lymph vessels begin in the cortex and they return the protein reabsorbed from the tubular fluid back to the blood.

The vasculature of the kidney is highly variable. Each kidney is usually supplied by a single artery, though multiple arteries are not uncommon. These can be a result of either renal artery branching or independent vessels branching off the aorta.

- The arteries branch into five **interlobar arteries** along the sides of the pyramids, which then divide into the **arcuate arteries** at the junction of the medulla and cortex
- The arcuate arteries then give rise to **inter-lobular arteries**
- The **afferent arterioles** feed into the glomeruli (Bowman's capsule) and drain into **efferent arterioles** (similar to portal blood vessels)
- In the cortex, which is the most highly vascularised part of the kidney, the efferent arterioles form a capillary network around the proximal tubules, known as the **peritubular capillaries**
- The juxtamedullary glomeruli give rise to the capillary networks known as the **vasa recta**, which eventually drain into the renal vein by forming tributaries
- The vasa recta, peritubular capillaries and the **loops of Henle** are involved in the **countercurrent exchange mechanism** responsible for urinary concentration

The ureters

Urine flows from the pelvis of the kidney through the ureters to the bladder and then out via the urethra. The ureters are about 25–30 cm long.

Nerve supply

The ureters receive both a sympathetic and parasympathetic supply via the spinal segments of the L1 and L2 nerve roots.

- The sympathetic supply is from the renal and intermesenteric plexus (upper ureter), the superior hypogastric plexus (middle ureter) and the inferior hypogastric (lower ureter)
- The parasympathetic vagal supply is via the coeliac plexus and the pelvic splanchnic nerves

Blood supply

The blood supply to the ureter comes from the renal, abdominal aorta, testicular or ovarian, common iliac, internal iliac, vesical and uterine arteries. The venous drainage is paired with the arterial supply, and the lymphatic drainage is to the lumbar, common and internal iliac and vesical nodes.

> ## Clinical insight
>
> The ureters are narrowed at three sites. – the pelviureteric junction, the pelvic brim and the ureteric orifice – making these the likely sites for obstruction by ureteric calculi.

The bladder and urethra

The bladder is a chamber for holding urine. It consists of a body in which urine collects, and a funnel-shaped bladder neck, which passes inferiorly into the urogenital triangle (the anterior perineum) and connects with the urethra. The external sphincter surrounds the junction of the bladder neck and the urethra. In the posterior wall of the bladder immediately above the bladder neck is the **trigone**, which has a smooth mucosa as opposed to the general **rugae** lining the rest of the bladder. The upper angles of the trigone mark the entry of the ureters and the lower the exit of the urethra.

The bladder has variable stretching ability as it consists of connective tissue and smooth muscle known as **detrusor**. Its unique structure enables it hold up to 500–1000 mL of urine comfortably.

Males have a longer urethra than females with valves between the bladder and the exit of the urethra. Abnormalities of the intravesical region are among the commonest causes of congenital renal disease in males.

> ## Clinical insight
>
> The muscles of the bladder distend as urine is drained into it. If bladder pressure exceeds the urethral sphincter resistance, incontinence develops.

Relations

- The bladder lies posterior to the pubic symphysis, anterior to the rectum in males and the vagina in females
- The superior surface is covered by the peritoneum
- In males the prostate surrounds the upper part of the urethra

> ## Clinical insight
>
> Vesicoureteric reflux should be excluded in young boys with bedwetting problems or recurrent urine infections. Left unchecked it can lead to scarring and irreversible damage to the kidneys.

Nerve supply

The bladder and urethra are supplied by S2–4 parasympathetic nerve fibres, which stimulate bladder emptying, vasodilation and penile erection. The sympathetic supply to the bladder arises from T10/11–L3 nerve root segments and their drive reduces bladder tone by inhibiting the parasympathetic effect. The bladder neck and proximal urethra are more richly innervated by sympathetic fibres, which act to facilitate their closure. This explains why α-blockers can induce incontinence or relieve the outflow obstruction in benign prostate hypertrophy. The bladder rests on the pelvic diaphragm, which is innervated by somatic motor neurones S2-4 that assist in voluntary contraction (**Table 1.1**).

The act of urinating (micturition) occurs through a complex coordinated stimulation of parasympathetic and inhibition of sympathetic tone. The act of voiding and its control is also dependent on the somatic nerve supply to the pelvic diaphragm and on the central nervous system.

Clinical insight

Females are more prone to urinary tract infections than males because of their relatively short urethra and its proximity to the anal opening.

	Sympathetic nerve supply	Parasympathetic nerve supply	Somatic nerve supply
Body of the bladder	T10/11–L3 (hypogastric nerves)	S2–4	–
Bladder trigone	T10/11–L3 (hypogastric nerves)	–	–
Bladder neck	T10/11–L3 (hypogastric nerves)	S2–4	–
External sphincter	–	S2–4	S2–4 (pudendal nerve)

Table 1.1 Innervation of the lower urinary tract.

Blood supply

The blood supply of the bladder and urethra comes from branches of the internal iliac arteries; the veins drain into the iliac internal veins. The lymphatic drainage is to the external, internal and sacral lymph nodes.

Histology of the urinary tract

A sagittal section of the renal tract reveals the parenchyma of the kidney; the outer dark brown **cortex** and the inner pale **medulla** and renal pelvis. The parenchyma is made up of interstitial tissue and **nephrons**, which consist of the **glomeruli** and their draining tubules (**Figure 1.5**). Each kidney contains over a million nephrons, although this number decreases with increasing age. This is known as a reduction in **nephron mass**, and explains why renal function decreases with age.

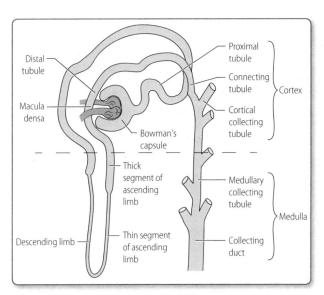

Figure 1.5 The nephron: the functional unit of the kidney.

The majority of the glomeruli are located in the cortex, with about 15% in the **juxtamedullary region**, the deepest region of the cortex. The medulla consists of dark, striated regions called the **pyramids**, which have apices known as **papillae**. The papillae project into the renal pelvis, which continues as the ureter (**Figure 1.3**).

Glomeruli

These are made up of tufts of vasculature (capillaries) contained within the cupped end of the renal tubule, known as **glomerular capsules** (or **Bowman's capsule**). The glomerular basement membrane (GBM) acts as the skeleton of the glomerular tuft and is lined by epithelial cells with projections forming filtration slits (**podocytes**) and interspersing phagocytic **mesangial cells**.

Tubules

The renal tubules are the small epithelial tubes making up the nephron that connect the glomerular capsules with the renal papillae. The capsule gives rise to the **proximal convoluted tubule** (PCT), the descending and ascending limbs of the loop of Henle, the **distal convoluted tubule** (DCT), which has an early convoluted segment, a short connecting segment and a late segment. Finally, the DCT becomes the **collecting duct** as it passes through the outer and inner medulla and opens at the tip of the renal papilla, draining filtrate into the renal pelvis.

Embryology of the urinary tract

During early development in males and females, both the urinary and genital ducts open out into the **cloaca**, the distal portion of the hindgut. The distal aspect of the excretory duct continues to be shared in males while in females the primitive part undergoes regression. The fetal urine passes into the **allantoic** or **amniotic fluid sac** from where it is reabsorbed. Interestingly, the kidney does not take on its excretory function until after birth even though it is fully developed by the 12th week. The kidney derives from the sequential development of the embryonic mesodermal kidney structures: **pronephros**, **mesonephros** and **metanephros** (**Figure 1.6**). The kidneys

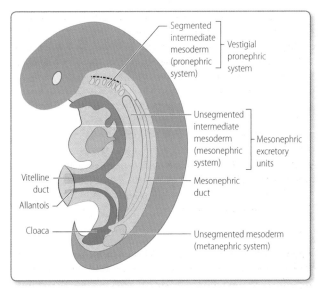

Figure 1.6 Relationship of the pronephros, mesonephros and metanephros in the development of the urogenital system.

develop from the metanephros, whereas the bladder and ureters develop from the **urogenital sinus**. In males, the prostate develops from an outgrowth of the urethral epithelium.

Clinical insight

Close development of the genital and urinary tract explains the relatively common association of genital and urinary tract malformations.

1.3 Physiology

Body fluids

The human body consists of 60% fluid in adult males, 50% in adult females and 75% in newborns. The body is divided into **extracellular** and **intracellular** fluid compartments. A 70 kg man would therefore have a total fluid content of approximately 42 L, with 28 L located in the intracellular and 14 L in the extracellular compartment. The extracellular fluid has 11 L as **interstitial fluid** and 3 L as **plasma**.

The constituents of the fluid are important for maintaining an optimum and steady physiological environment for cellular function. The main ions dissolved in the fluid (i.e. electrolytes) are sodium (Na^+), potassium (K^+), calcium (Ca^{2+}), magnesium (Mg^{2+}), chloride (Cl^-), hydrogen phosphate (HPO_4^{2-}) and hydrogen carbonate (HCO_3, also commonly known as bicarbonate). Sodium is the most abundant extracellular electrolyte while potassium is the main intracellular electrolyte.

Plasma osmolality is a measure of the body fluid/electrolyte balance and is normally between 275–295 mOsm/kg, i.e. milliosmoles of solute (electrolytes) per kilogram of solvent (water).

Kidney function

The kidneys have a central function in maintaining body fluid homeostasis. Their specific functions include:
- Excretion of metabolic waste products and foreign chemicals from the body
- Regulation of water, body electrolytes and fluid osmolality
- Regulation of acid-base balance
- Endocrine functions via specialised cells involved in the secretion, metabolism and excretion of hormones
- Blood pressure regulation

Guiding principle

The total number of nephrons a kidney has is fixed in utero. Once a nephron is lost it cannot be regenerated hence we all have a reduction in the number of nephrons with age, making a decline in renal function inevitable as we get older.

Urine formation

The purpose of urine formation is to excrete metabolic waste products and foreign chemicals. Urine formation starts by ultrafiltration of plasma (blood without red blood cells (RBCs)). This occurs in the glomerular capsules. Blood enters via the afferent arterioles and is then filtered through the basement membrane of the glomerular tufts in the glomerular capsule. Filtration is also influenced by the podocytes and mesangium.

Filtration is largely determined by the size of the molecules and the space between the podocyte foot processes known as slit diaphragms, which are around 30–40 nm in diameter. These are partially occluded by zipper-like structures so the actual spaces are even smaller. For example albumin has a molecular weight of 67 kDa and so does not pass through in normal physiological situations. Podocytes also affect filtration through their negative surface charge repelling negatively-charged molecules, discouraging their passage through the slits.

Mesangial cells fill the intercapillary spaces and regulate blood flow within the glomerular capillaries. Contraction of mesangia decreases GBM surface area, and therefore decreases the rate at which fluid is filtered by the glomeruli; the **glomerular filtration rate** (GFR).

Glomerular filtration rate

GFR can be estimated by comparing the amount of a specific chemical in plasma and urine that has a steady blood concentration, passes through the filtration slits unhindered, and is not reabsorbed or secreted by tubular cells. The rate is therefore the amount of the chemical in urine that came from a known amount in the blood, over time.

$$C_Y = U_Y \times V/P_Y$$

Where:
- C_Y is the renal clearance of substance 'y' (i.e. GFR)
- U_Y is the urine concentration
- V is the urine flow rate
- P_Y is the plasma concentration of substance 'y'

Factors affecting GFR   The major determinants of GFR are the:
- Renal blood flow and renal perfusion pressure
- Hydrostatic pressure difference between the tubule and the capillaries
- Surface area available for ultrafiltration

Renal blood flow   The blood supply to the kidneys is between 20% and 25% of cardiac output, i.e. approximately 1200 mL/min. Of this, renal plasma flow is about 660 mL/min, and 120 mL/min is filtered out of the blood and into the nephron. Ultimately, about 1.2 mL of this fluid is excreted as urine (1% of filtered load).

Renal blood flow is determined by the difference in pressure between the renal artery and the renal vein and is dependent on **total renal vascular resistance**. The renal vascular resistance is determined by the sum of the resistance in the arteries, arterioles, capillaries and veins.

$$\frac{\text{Renal}}{\text{blood flow}} = \frac{\text{(Renal artery pressure} - \text{Renal vein pressure)}}{\text{Total renal vascular resistance}}$$

The vascular resistance of these vessels is determined by the sympathetic nervous system, hormones including adrenaline, noradrenaline, endothelin, renin, angiotensin II, prostaglandins and local internal renal mechanisms. Sometimes external variables such as high glucose levels or high protein intake lead to increased renal blood flow.

Urinary excretion For any given substance, this is dependent on the GFR and is increased by tubular secretion but reduced by tubular reabsorption of the substance.

> ## Guiding principle
>
> Filtration = glomerular filtration rate × plasma concentration

$$\text{Urinary excretion} = \text{glomerular filtration} - \text{(tubular reabsorption} + \text{tubular secretion)}$$

Nitrogenous products such as urea, creatinine and urate are among the main metabolic products removed in urine. Urea is a breakdown product of amino acids, consisting of ammonia combined with carbon dioxide to make it less toxic. Urea excretion is partly dependent on dietary protein intake and liver function. Creatinine is a breakdown product of creatine phosphate, hence its concentration varies according to an individual's muscle bulk.

If a substance is freely filtered by the glomerulus and not reabsorbed or secreted, then its renal clearance will be equal to its GFR or the volume of plasma filtered per unit time. Very few substances meet these criteria. However, to obtain an accurate assessment of renal function substances such as inulin, iohexol and ^{51}Cr ethylenediaminetetraacetic acid (^{51}Cr EDTA) or ^{99m}Tc diethylene triamine pentaacetic acid (^{99m}Tc DTPA) are used.

Creatinine levels are routinely used to assess renal function but limitations include its variable tubular secretion in the proximal tubules. Urea is also used but has limitations.

Regulation of body fluid, osmolality and electrolyte concentration

Body fluid, osmolality and electrolyte concentration are regulated by the kidney through tubular reabsorption and secretion of sodium (Na), potassium (K), calcium (Ca), phosphate (PO_4), magnesium (Mg), chloride (Cl) and bicarbonate (HCO_3) (**Figures 1.7** and **1.8a–e**). The kidneys also regulate water balance and subsequently osmolality by controlling ion and water excretion in the tubules. The normal range for plasma osmolality is 275–299 mOsm/kg. This is maintained by a variety of feedback mechanisms.

> ### Clinical insight
>
> Limitations of using creatinine clearance and urea for assessing renal function include diet, muscle mass, ethnicity, gastrointestinal bleeds, high fevers, burns and drugs such as trimethoprim, tetracycline, corticosteroids and cimetidine.

> ### Clinical insight
>
> Renal regulation of blood sodium levels is a key function of the kidney as sodium is the main solute in extracellular fluid and has a major role in osmolality control.
>
> **Hypernatraemia** (increased plasma sodium concentration) is usually due to loss of water (e.g. diabetes insipidus).
>
> **Hyponatraemia** (low plasma sodium concentration) is common in sick patients, and is also found in the syndrome of inappropriate anti-diuretic hormone (SIADH) secretion. See Chapter 7 for more on causes and treatment.

The water balance influences plasma volume and has a direct effect on the blood pressure. The mechanism by which the kidney concentrates and dilutes the urine is largely dependent on the tubules.

Tubular reabsorption and secretion

PCT   The tubule arises from the glomerular capsule initially as the PCT, which is divided into segments **S1** and **S2**. The PCT is lined with cuboidal cells with multiple microvilli and is responsible for reabsorption of two thirds of the filtered salt,

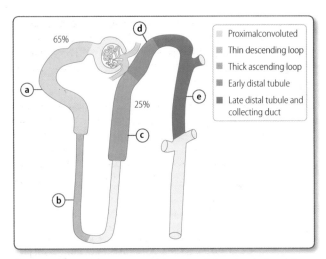

Figure 1.7 The nephron: secretion and absorption of electrolytes in the tubules. (a) proximal convoluted tubule, (b) thin descending loop of Henle, (c) thick ascending loop of Henle, (d) early distal tubule, (e) late distal tubule and collecting duct.

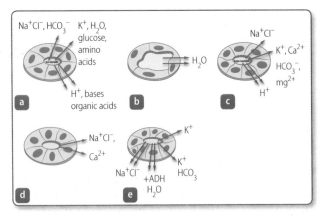

Figure 1.8 Secretion and absorption of electrolytes in the (a) proximal convoluted tubule, (b) thin descending loop of Henle, (c) thick ascending loop of Henle, (d) early distal tubule, and (e) late distal tubule and collecting duct. ADH, antidiuretic hormone.

water, and organic solutes such as amino acids and glucose. Sodium and water reabsorption are driven by osmosis whereas organic solute absorption is active and depends on co-transport channels involving ATPase. The S2 segment is followed by **S3**, the straight proximal tubule (PST).

Loop of Henle   The loop of Henle is the U-shaped part of the tubule, consisting of a descending and ascending limb. Its main function is to enable concentration of the urine. The descending loop is impermeable to salt but not water while the ascending loop is impermeable to water. This feature and the dense capillaries surrounding this part of the tubule enable the **countercurrent exchange mechanism** (also known as the countercurrent multiplication system):

1. Fluid leaving the ascending loop is hypo-osmolar: 100 mOsm/kg compared with that entering it (1000-1200 mOsm/kg)
2. The osmolality of the fluid at the bend of the loop is several times higher than that of the fluid entering it
3. The tissue interstitium in the cortex around the limbs of the loop has a much lower osmolality (100 mOsm/kg) than the osmolality of the tissue around the bend of the loop (1200 mOsm/kg) in the medulla

The third factor provides the optimal milieu for the collecting ducts, which pass from the cortex to the medulla, extracting as much water as possible, under the influence of anti-diuretic hormone (ADH). Finally, they drain into the renal pelvises.

> ### Guiding principle
>
> Desert animals like the marsupial mouse in Australia have highly developed countercurrent mechanisms with long loops of Henle, necessary in order to conserve as much fluid as possible.

DCT and collecting duct   The ascending loop of Henle and collecting duct are connected by the DCT. The cells lining the DCT are dense in mitochondria and the ion exchange occurring in this segment of the tubule is largely hormone-driven by parathyroid hormone (Ca reabsorbed, PO_4 excreted), aldosterone (Na reabsorbed, K excreted) and atrial natriuretic peptide (Na excretion).

By the end of the DCT, the filtrate has only 3% of its water content compared to the capsular filtrate. Osmosis is responsible for the resorption of 97.9% of the glomerular filtrate water entering the convoluted tubules and collecting ducts.

Acid–base balance

Similar to the kidney's role in regulating osmolality, extracellular fluid and electrolyte balance, it is also responsible – in conjunction with the lungs – for maintaining homeostasis of the plasma pH. The kidneys are mainly responsible for long-term adjustments; they achieve this through hydrogen ion excretion to bring about a steady state. Chapter 8 deals with the mechanism for acid transport in different parts of nephron, and clinical and biochemical features of acid–base derangement as well as the defence mechanisms to prevent abrupt changes in pH.

Secretion, metabolism and excretion of hormones
Renin

Renin is a 406 amino acid enzyme that is central to blood pressure control (**Figure 1.9**). It is synthesised and stored in the **juxtaglomerular apparatus** (JGA) of the kidneys (**Figure 1.10**). The JGA is formed by part of the ascending loop of Henle, where it turns to become the DCT and passes close to its own Bowman's capsule, coming in to contact with the afferent and efferent arterioles. The DCT cells in this area are known as the **macula densa** and the afferent arteriole wall cells as granular cells. Renin is released by the granular cells when:

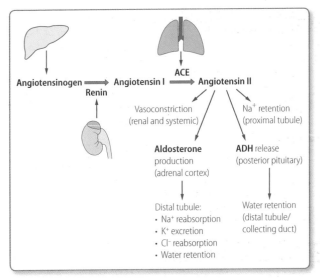

Figure 1.9 The renin–angiotensin–aldosterone system. ACE, angiotensin–converting enzyme. ADH, antidiuretic hormone.

- A fall in ECF volume is detected by peripheral baroreceptors, causing increased sympathetic activity to granular cells
- The macula densa cells sense a decrease in [Na] within the DCT and secrete prostaglandin, stimulating granular cell release of renin
- A fall in ECF decreases pressure in the afferent arterioles, detected by granular cells.

The effects of renin on blood pressure are by its actions on **angiotensinogen**, an α_2 globulin produced by the liver:

- Renin converts angiotensinogen to **angiotensin I** (a decapeptide), which is then converted by angiotensin–converting enzyme (ACE) to **angiotensin II** (an octapeptide)
- Angiotensin II acts to maintain vascular pressure by causing vasoconstriction, and by stimulating aldosterone production from the zona glomerulosa of the adrenals

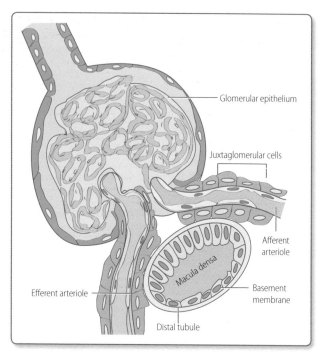

Figure 1.10 The juxtaglomerular apparatus.

- Angiotensin II at higher concentrations causes vasoconstriction of the afferent arteriole, leading to a reduction in GFR. At lower concentrations, it causes vasoconstriction of the efferent arteriole, helping to maintain GFR by elevating intraglomerular pressure.

Erythropoietin

The kidney produces 80% of the body's erythropoietin, the liver synthesises the rest. Hypoxia stimulates its prostaglandin-mediated production by mesangial and tubular cells, which leads to increased erythropoiesis in the bone marrow. Release of erythropoietin is also enhanced by catecholamines acting via β-receptors.

Vitamin D

Vitamin D is a steroid hormone synthesised in the skin, and then hydroxylated in the liver (**25-hydroxycholecalciferol**) and in the kidney (**1, 25 dihydroxycholecalciferol**). It is essential for bone and teeth mineralisation and acts by enhancing absorption of calcium and phosphate from the gut (**Figure 1.11**). It is counter-regulated by the parathyroid gland hence problems with its production can lead to parathyroid disease (see Chapter 4).

Clinical insight

Patients with renal disease have reduced erythropoietin production and as a consequence develop hypochromic normochromic anaemia. Erythropoietin produced by recombinant DNA is often used to replace the natural form in patients with chronic kidney disease to correct the anaemia.

Patients with chronic kidney disease (CKD) show a reduced response to recombinant erythropoietin in the presence of sepsis, iron, folate and vitamin B12 deficiency, malignancy, bleeding and parathyroid disease.

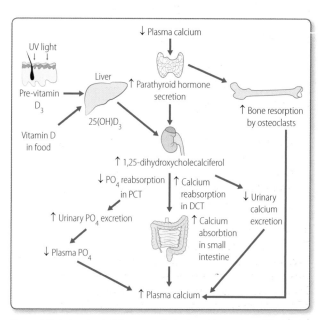

Figure 1.11 Active vitamin D has a central role alongside parathyroid hormone in calcium regulation.

Clinical insight

The inhibition of prostaglandin synthesis in the kidney by non-steroidal anti-inflammatory drugs (NSAIDs) such as ibuprofen may have no effect in the normal individual but in patients with volume depletion it can cause a profound fall in the GFR.

Prostaglandins and other arachidonate metabolites

Arachidonates are complex lipids that are synthesised by most of the cells in the body. Those peculiar to the kidney include the prostaglandins (PGs) PGE2, PGI2, PGF2a, PGD2 and thromboxane A2.

They are produced by cortical and medullary interstitial cells and also by the epithelial cells of the collecting ducts. PGs have a vasodilatory role and can also contribute to diuresis and naturesis.

Endothelins

Endothelins are a family of peptides that act on the renal vasculature to induce potent vasoconstriction. Endothelins 1–3 are produced by the mesangial cells, and the afferent and efferent arterioles. They have both autocrine and paracrine effects, and induce contraction and vasoconstriction. This may lead to alteration in renal blood flow and GFR particularly in pathological conditions such as contrast nephropathy and congestive heart failure. Their exact homeostatic function in normal physiology is less clear.

Purines

Purines produced by the kidneys include adenosine and adenosine triphosphate (ATP). They are locally produced and appear to act both on tubules, affecting water and sodium reabsorption, and on the arterioles, causing vasoconstriction. Their precise physiological role is still being explored.

Gluconeogenic enzymes

Most gluconeogenesis (synthesis of glucose) is carried out by the liver. However, the renal cortex has gluconeogenic enzymes and, in situations such as prolonged fasting, can contribute up to 50% of the body's production. It produces glucose from lactate, glycerol and glutamine as opposed to glycogen, the predominant source for glucose production by the liver. Glucose production by the kidney is partly regulated by insulin and catecholamines.

Clinical essentials

2.1 Common symptoms and how to take a history

This section outlines the salient features to cover in the history. Patients with kidney disease will often have few symptoms and present late in the course of their disease. Unlike other specialties, there are few cardinal features of kidney disease, but certain symptoms and signs can indicate a particular underlying aetiology. A systematic approach involving direct questioning should elicit all the relevant information required in making a diagnosis.

Common symptoms
Urinary abnormalities

Reduced urine output   Occasionally patients report reduced urine output or not passing any urine, which is most often indicative of obstructive urological pathology. In males, this is most commonly due to prostatic disease. Ask about previous obstructive symptoms such as:
- Difficulty passing urine
- Poor urinary stream
- Urinary dribbling

Obstruction can also occur due to abdominal or pelvic **malignancy**, caused by either locally advanced disease or **ureteric strictures** following radiotherapy. This may be evident from the history. Occasionally, the obstruction is due to retroperitoneal fibrosis.

Little or no urine output in the acute setting can also be due to **acute tubular necrosis** (ATN) or **bilateral vascular occlusion**. As a symptom in the context of chronic disease, it is less helpful as patients are more likely to maintain urine output even with a low glomerular filtration rate (GFR).

Dysuria   This is a burning sensation felt while passing urine, and is a common symptom of urinary tract infections (UTIs).

Macroscopic haematuria   The presence of visible blood in the urine can be a sign of kidney stones or UTIs, both also associated with pain.

Painless episodes indicate bleeding somewhere along the urinary tract. Initially, urological **malignancy** should be excluded in those with risk factors, i.e. older age (over 40 years) and smokers. In younger patients, and in those where urological pathology has been excluded, it can indicate **glomerular bleeding**, particularly if accompanied by hypertension and reduced renal function.

Episodes of macroscopic haematuria characteristically occur with **IgA nephropathy** during an intercurrent infection, which is typically respiratory in nature.

Frothy urine   This can indicate significant **proteinuria** and should prompt evaluation for proteinuria. It is often reported by patients who have previously experienced **nephrotic syndrome** and recognise the symptom as a recurrence of their disease.

Loin pain

Pain in the region of the kidneys is described as loin pain. Unilateral or bilateral loin pain often occurs with **infection**. It is indicative of **pyelonephritis** when accompanied by fever and haematuria.

More severe, colicky loin pain can indicate a **renal stone**. Other symptoms of a stone include:
- Passage of gritty urine, as small particles of the stone are passed
- Haematuria
- Pain on micturition as the stone is passed

Leg swelling

Bilateral leg swelling suggests **oedema** and is a relatively common symptom. It can be due to volume overload secondary to cardiac, liver or renal failure. **Nephrotic syndrome** should be considered and this symptom should prompt urinalysis for proteinuria. Absence of proteinuria excludes nephrotic syndrome as a diagnosis.

Uraemic symptoms

These symptoms often come on insidiously and indicate **severe renal impairment**, whatever the underlying cause. It is important to ask about them directly as often patients will not volunteer these symptoms due to their slow onset. The main uraemic symptoms are:

- Tiredness
- Loss of appetite
- Weight loss
- Metallic taste
- Nausea
- Vomiting

Haemoptysis

Haemoptysis is the coughing up of blood. It is seen with **pulmonary oedema** when it tends to occur as pink, frothy sputum. Haemoptysis should also raise the possibility of pulmonary haemorrhage secondary to **vasculitis** or **Goodpasture's disease**, prompting appropriate investigation for these conditions.

Haemoptysis can be due to primary respiratory disease such as **pneumonia** or **lung malignancy** which may have secondary kidney pathology. Acute kidney injury (AKI) due to ATN can occur in any infection including pneumonia, and nephrotic syndrome due to membranous nephropathy can be secondary to a solid organ tumour.

Rash

There are a variety of rashes that may be a presentation of a disease with renal involvement. Types of rash important in renal disease are discussed in section 2.2.

Arthralgia

Arthralgia or pain in the joints is a common symptom in patients with **systemic lupus erythematosus** (SLE) and **vasculitis**. It can present in any joint, but typically occurs in the small joints.

Pain in the large joints characteristically occurs in **Henoch–Schönlein purpura**, especially when accompanied by a vasculitic rash on the buttocks.

Ear, nose and throat (ENT) symptoms

Symptoms involving the ear, nose or throat (e.g. a blocked nose, sinusitis or nasal polyps) typically occur in **granulomatosis with polyangiitis** (previously called Wegener granulomatosis) and is due to granulomatous disease along the ENT tract.

The symptoms may have been present for many years and can pre-date the kidney disease. They should be asked about directly as they may not be volunteered.

Past history

A past history of recurrent urinary infections, particularly as a child, should be asked about as this would be compatible with **reflux nephropathy**.

Family history

The patient should be asked whether any family members have kidney problems or are known to have blood or protein in the urine.

- The most common genetic renal disease is **adult polycystic kidney disease** (PKD), which is inherited in an autosomal pattern
- Less common inherited renal disorders include **Fabry** and **Alport diseases**; both are most commonly X-linked recessive and so males are more likely to be affected. The latter is associated with sensorineural deafness, which may also be a feature in the family
- A few **glomerular diseases** have a non-mendelian pattern of inheritance, e.g. some types of focal segmental glomerulosclerosis (FSGS)

Drug history

A detailed current and historical drug history should be taken. The timeline of when the drugs were taken in relation to the presentation of kidney disease may be relevant.

The history should include prescription and non-prescribed drugs. Particular note should be made about the use of non-steroidal anti-inflammatory drugs (NSAIDs), antibiotics and herbal remedies. Some examples of known nephrotoxic herbal remedies include Chinese herbal aristocholic acid (a known cause of kidney failure), and some West African herbal remedies (which contain NSAIDs and can cause renal impairment).

Guiding principle

Presenting symptoms:

- Urinary abnormalities: reduced urine output, haematuria, urinary tract infections, obstructive urinary symptoms
- Uraemic symptoms
- Systemic symptoms, e.g. rash, arthralgia (vasculitis, systemic lupus erythematosus), ENT symptoms (e.g. granulomatosis with polyangiitis)

Past history: recurrent urinary tract infections, especially as a child (reflux nephropathy)

Drug history (to identify potentially nephrotoxic agents):

- Current and historical
- Antibiotics, chemotherapy agents, NSAIDs
- Recreational
- Alternative and herbal remedies (especially Chinese herbal medicines)

Family history: kidney disease or blood/protein in urine

2.2 Common signs and how to examine the patient

A complete examination of all systems should be undertaken, particularly as some diseases that affect the kidneys are secondary to systemic illness. A systematic, logical approach will ensure that all systems are covered.

A typical examination starts with general inspec-

Guiding principle

Keep the order in which body systems are examined constant so that, over time, it becomes second nature. Identification of signs can then become the focus.

tion, followed by the examination of each system, traditionally starting with cardiac and then respiratory. Working down the body, the abdomen is then examined, followed by the nervous system. The following sections highlight the common signs of renal disease seen in each system.

General inspection
A high temperature

A temperature of over 37°C should raise the possibility of **infections** such as infective endocarditis, and appropriate microbiological investigations including blood cultures should be done. Inflammatory conditions including vasculitis, SLE and allergic tubulointerstitial nephritis should also be considered.

Skin colour

A lemon-yellow tinge to the skin may occur in **uraemia**. Pallor of the conjunctiva indicates **anaemia**, a complication of renal impairment.

Skin rashes

A number of rashes can occur in different diseases that affect the kidney:

- Vasculitic rash: a palpable, non-blanching purpuric rash seen mainly in the extremities is typical of a vasculitic rash and can occur in primary **vasculitides** and **infective endocarditis**
- Purpuric rash: a purpuric rash on the buttocks, particularly in young males, associated with arthralgia is consistent with **Henoch–Schönlein purpura**
- Butterfly rash: an erythematous butterfly-shaped rash across the cheeks of the face is typical of **SLE**
- Photosensitive rash: an erythematous photosensitive rash in sun-exposed areas can also occur in **SLE**
- Erythematous maculo-papular rash: an erythematous maculo-papular rash all over the body can occur in **tubulointerstitial nephritis**
- Livedo reticularis: blue toes and livedo reticularis can occur in **atheroembolic disease**

Nails

The presence of nail fold infarcts and/or splinter haemorrhages should raise the suspicion of **infective endocarditis** or **vasculitis**.

Joints

Inflammation, particularly in the small joints, often occurs in **SLE**, and this diagnosis should be considered when this is accompanied by a rash, particularly in young females of Afro-Caribbean or Asian origin. Inflammation in the joints can also occur with **vasculitis**.

Hair

Alopecia is loss of hair from the head and body. Its presence should raise suspicion of **SLE**. The hair loss typically occurs in patches, while complete hair loss from the scalp and other areas of the body is rare.

Cardiovascular system
High blood pressure

Due to the kidney's key role in blood pressure homeostasis, a high blood pressure of >140/80 mm Hg is commonly seen in patients with kidney disease, particularly in glomerular or vascular disorders. The pathogenesis varies depending on the type and duration of disease (**Table 2.1**).

Elevated jugular venous pressure

The jugular venous pressure (JVP) is an indirect measure of venous pressure obtained by observing the internal jugular vein:

> ## Clinical insight
>
> Examination of the JVP:
> - Examine the patient at 45°
> - Ensure the patient's neck is relaxed
> - It is easier to visualise the JVP from the side, i.e. along the surface of the sternocleidomastoid muscle, rather than looking at it directly
>
> Characteristics of the JVP:
> - Position: it is visualised between the two heads of the sternocleidomastoid
> - Character: It is a double waveform, non-pulsatile and compressible
> - It moves with respiration, specifically downward with inspiration
> - It moves with position, specifically downward when the patient sits upright and upward when the patient is more prone
> - Hepatojugular reflux: it moves upwards when the liver is pressed gently

- A normal JVP is visible at the level of the clavicle when the patient is at a 45° angle
- An **elevated JVP** is seen above this level and suggests volume overload. It can also be elevated for other reasons in patients with heart and lung disease

Type of kidney disease	Pathogenesis of hypertension
Acute glomerular, e.g. post-infectious glomerulonephritis	Fluid and sodium retention
Acute vascular, e.g. vasculitis	Activation of the renin–angiotensin system
Chronic kidney disease	Fluid and sodium retention Activation of renin–angiotensin system Enhanced sympathetic activity Impaired nitric oxide synthesis
Renovascular	Reduced renal perfusion Activation of renin–angiotensin system

Table 2.1 Pathogenesis of hypertension in different types of kidney disease.

- The JVP will not be visible if the patient is volume depleted, but it may be seen with the hepatojugular reflux or when the patient lies more prone

Pericardial rub

A pericardial rub is a scratchy noise heard on auscultation of the heart in addition to the heart sounds. Its quality changes with respiration and position and it is best heard in the left midsternal region with the patient leaning forward. It indicates inflammation of the pericardium, which has a number of causes. In the context of severe renal impairment it can be due to uraemia (**uraemic pericarditis**). This is rare and worth noting as an indication for dialysis.

New murmur

A murmur that has not been previously detected may suggest **infective endocarditis**, particularly when present with other signs such as a high temperature, vasculitic phenomenon (e.g. splinter haemorrhages) and risk factors such as recent dental treatment or poor dentition. It should prompt three sets of blood cultures to isolate the microorganism.

To investigate the possibility of **glomerular disease** associated with endocarditis, urinalysis should be carried out. Absence of blood and protein on dipstick testing excludes this diagnosis. Complement levels should also be assessed; low complement levels can occur in infective endocarditis particularly with associated glomerular disease but normal levels do not exclude these diagnoses.

Peripheral pitting oedema

Oedema is the accumulation of fluid in body tissues, often accumulating in the legs and seen as leg swelling. Pitting refers to the indentation of the skin that occurs on pressing the skin for up to 30 seconds. It is important to differentiate pitting from non-pitting oedema as the likely causes differ:

- *Non-pitting* oedema is not associated with kidney disease
- *Pitting* oedema often occurs in volume overload when there is accumulation of fluid in the tissues. Its presence suggests **nephrotic syndrome** and should prompt urinalysis. It can also occur in the context of renal impairment whatever the underlying cause

Renal bruit

A bruit is a systolic noise heard with a stethoscope over an artery. It is a harsh, machinery- type sound due to turbulent flow in the arteries. A renal bruit is heard in the flank regions and may indicate **renal artery stenosis**. This should prompt examination of the peripheral pulses and auscultation for bruits elsewhere, e.g. the carotid arteries and abdominal aorta. Absence of peripheral pulses and presence of bruits indicate the likelihood of **atherosclerotic disease**.

Respiratory system
End-inspiratory crackles

Bilateral crackles in the lung fields may indicate **pulmonary oedema**, especially if accompanied by other signs of volume overload such as an elevated JVP. Pink, frothy sputum can occur with pulmonary oedema. **Pulmonary haemorrhage** should be considered when bilateral crackles are heard in the context of haemoptysis and renal impairment. Patients are generally very unwell and often hypoxic with respiratory failure.

Abdomen
Large kidneys
Normal-sized kidneys are barely ballotable in a slim patient. Large, ballotable kidneys most commonly occur in adult **PKD**. This can be confirmed by renal ultrasound.

A palpable bladder
The bladder is examined in the suprapubic region. A bladder that is detectable by palpation or percussion indicates it contains at least 500 mL. This can suggest urinary outflow obstruction, most commonly seen with **prostatic disease** in males. It is often easily reversed by insertion of a catheter; drainage of a large residual volume confirms the diagnosis. Further management includes examination of the prostate and measurement of prostatic serum antigen (PSA).

Nervous system
Confusion
Acute confusion or delirium as well as drowsiness can occur with **uraemia**. These can be indications for renal replacement therapy.

Confusion, fits and upper motor neurone signs may occur due to cerebral involvement in **SLE**.

Peripheral neuropathy
If a secondary cause of kidney disease is suspected, a thorough neurological examination should be undertaken. Mononeuritis multiplex is the sequential involvement of multiple, single nerves (both sensory and motor components), and can occur in vasculitis and diabetes mellitus. Peripheral neuropathy, like nephropathy, is a microvascular complication of diabetes mellitus.

Eyes

Diabetic retinopathy   In patients with diabetes mellitus, the presence of diabetic retinopathy makes nephropathy much more likely. If diabetic retinopathy is absent, a diagnosis other than diabetic nephropathy should be considered.

Hypertensive retinopathy   If the blood pressure is very high and accelerated phase hypertension is suspected, there are likely to be retinal hypertensive changes. Mild changes include fibrotic arterioles (with a white/"silver-wiring" appearance) and arteriovenous nipping, which represent grade 1 and 2 changes, respectively. More severe changes typically are flame haemorrhages and cotton wool spots, which represent oedema, and swelling of the optic disc (papilloedema).

2.3 Investigations

This section covers the commonly used tests to investigate and manage renal disease:
- Blood tests
- Urine tests
- Radiology
- Histopathology

Blood tests
Biochemistry

Urea and electrolytes   High serum urea and creatinine concentrations indicate renal impairment. In most cases of kidney disease, these tests would already have been done.

Estimation of the GFR gives a measure of the number of functioning nephrons. The most common method is measurement of serum creatinine concentration. Creatinine rises exponentially with increasing severity of renal impairment. Hence, when creatinine is normal, small rises indicate larger decreases in GFR compared with the same amount of rise when the creatinine concentration is high.

The Modification of Diet in Renal Disease (MDRD) study equation, based on the serum creatinine and other variables such as age, is used to estimate GFR. Its validation and now routine use by many laboratories has improved early diagnosis and categorisation of chronic kidney disease (CKD) (see Chapter 4).

Clinical insight

Serum creatinine and the MDRD equation can only be used reliably in patients with stable kidney disease and not in AKI. With AKI, the GFR (and creatinine levels) may change over a period of hours.

Electrolyte abnormalities can occur as a complication of renal impairment, most commonly **hyperkalaemia** and **metabolic acidosis** (indicated by low bicarbonate). Other electrolyte abnormalities such as **hypokalaemia** may indicate a primary renal tubular abnormality and should prompt appropriate investigations (see Chapter 7).

C-reactive protein   A high c-reactive protein (CRP) is usually due to **infection**, but can also be due to inflammatory conditions such as **vasculitis**. If there is no obvious infection, consider inflammatory conditions as well as a chronic or occult infection such as infective endocarditis. The absence of blood and protein on urinalysis excludes renal vasculitis.

Albumin   A low albumin level (<30 g/L) raises the possibility of **nephrotic syndrome**. This is due, in part, to the urinary loss of protein. Due to changes in capillary permeability and oncotic pressure, albumin concentration can drop quickly in the sick patient (e.g. severe sepsis) without significant proteinuria.

Bone profile   Renal impairment causes typical abnormalities of serum calcium and phosphate concentrations:
- Hyperphosphotaemia occurs as the kidneys are less able to excrete phosphate
- Hypocalcaemia results from decreased kidney hydroxylation of 25-hydroxy vitamin D into the active form of calcitriol (1,25 hydroxy vitamin D)

Hyperphosphataemia, reduced active vitamin D (1,25 hydroxy vitamin D) and hypocalcaemia stimulate the parathyroid gland, and parathyroid hormone (PTH) concentrations rise in renal impairment. This can take weeks to months and so a high PTH level suggests that renal impairment has been present for some time.

Clinical insight

High calcium is unusual and should be investigated for its cause (e.g. myeloma).

Haemoglobin   Normocytic anaemia is a common finding in renal disease, due to a lack of erythropoietin production. Other causes of anaemia include:

- Normocytic anaemia: myeloma, vasculitis
- Haemolytic anaemia: SLE, microangiopathic haemolytic anaemia
- Microcytic anaemia: chronic blood loss from pulmonary haemorrhage

White cell count   A high white cell count (WCC) commonly indicates **infection** but can occur in other **inflammatory** conditions. The differential blood cell count should also be considered. Eosinophilia can occur in **tubulointerstitial nephritis** and **atheroembolic disease**, and is a diagnostic criterion for **Churg–Strauss vasculitis**. Neutrophilia can occur in other types of **vasculitis**.

Platelets   Thrombocytopenia (a low platelet level) typically occurs in **microangiopathic haemolytic anaemia**. A blood film should be requested to assess for typical findings of red cell fragments. There may also be low complement concentrations and a history of diarrhoea in the setting of **haemolytic uraemic syndrome**.

Low platelet levels also occur in **disseminated intravascular coagulopathy** (DIC), which often occurs as a result of overwhelming sepsis or bleeding. Low fibrinogen, high fibrin degradation products and long coagulation times are other features of DIC.

Immunological tests

A number of immunological assays should be considered to further investigate renal disease, especially when there is blood and/or protein present in the urine (**Table 2.2**). These, along with other blood tests of virology, complement concentrations and serum electrophoresis, constitute the 'acute renal screen'.

Antineutrophil cytoplasm antibody   Antineutrophil cytoplasm antibodies (ANCA) are autoantibodies that bind cytoplasmic antigens within neutrophils and are associated with vasculitis. There are two types of test for ANCA in serum:

Investigation	Description
c-ANCA (PR3)	Positive in 90% patients with active granulomatosis with polyangiitis
p-ANCA (MPO)	Positive in 60% patients with microscopic polyangitis and 30% patients with Churg-Strauss syndrome
Anti-GBM	Positive in anti-GBM (Goodpasture) disease
ANA	Positive in 90% patients with active SLE. Sensitive but not specific for SLE
Anti-dsDNA	Positive in 50% patients with active SLE, specific to SLE
Complement concentrations C3 and C4	Low levels in: • Post infectious GN • Mesangiocapillary GN • Immune complex GN, e.g. SLE, cryoglobulinaemia
Cryoglobulins	Presence associated with type 1 mesangiocapillary GN and hepatitis C infection
Viral serology: Hepatitis B, C and HIV	Can be associated with glomerular disease: • HIV: FSGS (nephrotic syndrome) • Hepatitis B: membranous (nephrotic syndrome), PAN • Hepatitis C: MCGN
Serum electrophoresis	Paraprotein suggests myeloma

Table 2.2 The 'acute renal screen': blood tests commonly used to investigate the cause of renal disease. ANA, antinuclear antibody . anti-GBM, antiglomerular basement membrane. c-ANCA, cytoplasmic antineutrophil cytoplasm antibody. dsDNA, double-stranded deoxyribonucleic acid. FSGS, focal segmental glomerulosclerosis. GN, glomerulonephritis. HIV, human immunodeficiency virus. MCGN, mesangiocapillary glomerulonephritis. MPO, myeloperoxidase. p-ANCA, perinuclear antineutrophil cytoplasm antibody. PR3, proteinase-3. SLE, systemic lupus erythematosus. PAN, polyarteritis nodosa.

- **Immunofluorescence** involves incubating the patient's serum with neutrophils and identifying whether ANCA binds to them. The presence is detected by a fluorescent-labelled antibody that subsequently binds to any patient-derived antibody bound to the neutrophil. There are two types of ANCA, defined by where in the neutrophil the patient's antibody binds: c-ANCA (**Figure 2.1**) indicates the antibody binds in the cytoplasm of the neutrophil; and p-ANCA (**Figure 2.2**) indicates that it binds in the perinuclear region of the neutrophil

- **Enzyme-linked immunoassay (ELISA)** detects the specific antigen in the neutrophil to which the antibody in the patient's serum binds. In the context of vasculitis, c-ANCA and p-ANCA detected by immunofluorescence are associated with antibodies directed to the antigens proteinase-3 (PR3) and myeloperoxidase (MPO), respectively, detected by ELISA

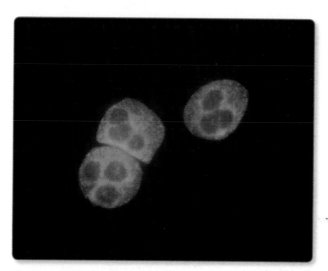

Figure 2.1 Cytoplasmic staining pattern by immunofluorescence of positive c-ANCA (cytoplasmic antineutrophil cytoplasmic antibody). (Courtesy of the Protein Reference Unit, St Georges Hospital, London)

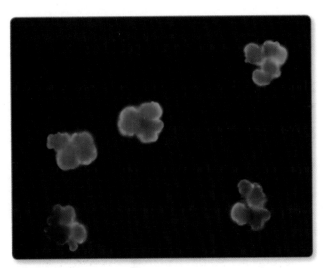

Figure 2.2 Perinuclear staining pattern by immunofluorescence of positive p-ANCA (perinuclear antineutrophil cytoplasmic antibody). (courtesy of Protein Reference Unit, St Georges Hospital)

Of the two methods, immunofluorescence is more sensitive but ELISA is more specific. Thus, ideally the two should be used together with the former for screening and the latter for confirmation of a positive ANCA.

Antibodies directed to other proteins (e.g. elastase, lysozyme) can also bind to neutrophils and lead to a positive ANCA test by immunofluorescence, particularly with a perinuclear pattern of staining. However, ANCA detection by ELISA would be negative. This 'false-positive' ANCA can occur in patients with antinuclear antibodies (ANA) and in chronic inflammatory conditions.

Clinical insight

In the setting of a positive ANCA by immunofluorescence, but negative ANCA by ELISA, a diagnosis of vasculitis is unlikely, and other causes for a false-positive ANCA should be sought.

Antiglomerular basement membrane (GBM) antibody   Anti-GBM antibody is an autoantibody directed against an antigen on the glomerular basement membrane. It is pathognomonic for **anti-GBM disease** (Goodpasture disease), in which the antibody binds to its target in the kidney and sometimes in the lungs, leading to a crescentic glomerulonephritis and pulmonary haemorrhage.

Antinuclear antibody   Antinuclear antibodies (ANA) are autoantibodies directed against the contents of the nucleus. A high titre is indicative of autoimmune diseases such as **SLE**, **Sjögren's disease** and **scleroderma**.

Double-stranded DNA (dsDNA) **antibody** is a subtype of ANA directed against dsDNA. It is highly specific for **SLE** and titre levels often correlate with disease activity.

Complement concentrations   The complement system is part of the innate immune system and consists of the classical, alternative and mannose-binding pathways. The components of the pathway are small blood proteins including C3 and C4, which are the ones commonly measured.

In the context of kidney disease, particularly when glomerular disease is suspected, measurement of complement levels is helpful as relatively few conditions are associated with low concentrations (see Table 2.2).

Virology
Hepatitis B and **C** viruses and the **human immunodeficiency virus** (HIV) can cause glomerular lesions and should be evaluated as part of investigation into the underlying cause of renal disease, especially if risk factors are present. Typically:
- HIV causes **FSGS**, which presents as **nephrotic syndrome**, mainly in Afro-Caribbeans
- Hepatitis B causes **membranous nephropathy** (nephrotic syndrome) and occasionally **polyarteritis nodosa**
- Hepatitis C is associated with a **type 1 mesangiocapillary glomerulonephritis** and cryoglobulinaemia

Viral serology for these infections should also be done if the patient is likely to need renal replacement therapy. Positive serology for any of these infections indicates that the patient and, in some places, haemodialysis machine need to be isolated to minimise the risk of cross-infection.

Serum protein electrophoresis   Serum electrophoresis should be done, particularly in older patients with kidney disease, to detect **myeloma**. It can present with either chronic or acute kidney impairment, often with no other symptoms.

Urine tests
Urine dipstick
Urine dipstick should be performed to identify the possibility of **glomerular disease**, which is indicated by the presence of significant proteinuria (3+) and/or haematuria. Absence of blood and protein makes glomerular disease extremely unlikely.

Little or no proteinuria with renal impairment suggests a non-glomerular pathology such as **ATN**, **tubulointerstitial nephritis** or **vascular** pathology.

Microalbuminuria
A small amount of albumin detected in the urine is an early sign of **diabetic nephropathy** but is not detected on urine dipstick tests. Urine should therefore be sent for an albumin:creatinine ratio (ACR) analysis to detect microalbuminuria (>30 mg/mmol).

Urine protein:creatine ratio
If protein is detected on dipstick, the amount of proteinuria present should be quantified. A one-off urine sample, ideally a first morning sample, is sent for protein:creatinine ratio analysis. This method has been validated and has advantages over 24-hour urine collection in terms of accuracy of collection and patient reliability.

Bence Jones protein
A test for urinary Bence Jones proteins should be performed in the elderly and when **myeloma** is suspected.

Urine microscopy
Microscopy should be done by an experienced person and is useful as there are characteristic findings specific to certain pathologies:

- Dysmorphic red cells and red cell casts indicates **glomerular pathology**
- White cell casts and eosinophils suggests **tubulointerstitial nephritis**
- Crystals are sometimes seen and are associated with certain **drugs**, e.g. indinavir, paraformaldehyde.

Radiology

The imaging techniques used to investigate renal disease are summarised in **Table 2.3**.

Assessment	Radiological test
Renal size and structure	Ultrasound scan CT (with contrast if possible) for more detail MRI can also be used
Obstruction	Ultrasound scan Dynamic isotope scan to identify functional obstruction CT (with contrast if possible) to identify cause
Stones	Plain film (initial test) Ultrasound scan Non-contrast CT (gold standard)
Recurrent urinary tract infections	Pre- and postmicturition ultrasound scan Micturating cystourethrogram
Renal scarring	DMSA scan
Split function	Dynamic isotope scan DMSA scan can be used
Renal artery stenosis	Doppler Magnetic resonance angiography Renal angiography (gold standard)
? Polyarteritis nodosa	Renal angiography

Table 2.3 Imaging techniques used to assess renal disease. CT, computed tomography. DMSA, dimercaptosuccinic acid. MRI, magnetic resonance imaging.

Plain X-ray

A plain X-ray of the kidneys, ureters and bladder (KUB) is not usually performed to investigate renal disease, except as an initial test for the detection of kidney stones in a patient with suggestive symptoms. It will identify calcium-containing stones (approximately 80% of all stones) but will miss small stones and all radiolucent stones.

Ultrasound scanning

Renal ultrasound scanning should be done in most patients with renal impairment to identify obstructive uropathy, assess the size of kidneys and identify structural abnormalities and asymmetry. It can also evaluate bladder emptying by assessing pre- and postmicturition volumes.

- Small kidneys (<10 cm) with thin cortices (<1 cm) indicate **chronic kidney disease**
- Large kidneys (>12 cm) suggest an infiltrative process such as **amyloidosis** or **lymphoma** as well as **HIV nephropathy**, although further evaluation for a definitive diagnosis is required

> ### Clinical insight
>
> Ultrasound is highly operator-dependent and evaluation is difficult in large or overweight patients.

Doppler ultrasound

This is useful to evaluate renal vascular flow and identify **renal artery stenosis, renal vein thrombosis, reduced renal perfusion** and **renal infarction**.

Computed tomography

Computed tomography (CT) of the kidneys, ureters and bladder (CT KUB) is useful to evaluate the anatomy and structure of the renal tract in more detail than ultrasound. It is used to identify the cause of **obstruction**, further evaluate renal masses, including distinction of complex from simple **cysts**, and stage renal **tumours**. The use of radioiodine contrast is preferable but should be considered with caution in those with significant renal impairment.

Non-contrast helical CT KUB is the gold standard for evaluation of **renal stones** and will detect stones missed on plain radiograph.

Magnetic resonance imaging

Magnetic resonance imaging (MRI) can be used for evaluation of **renovascular disease** and to identify **renal vein thrombosis**, although gadolinium (a MRI contrast agent) is contraindicated in patients with estimated GFR <30 mL/min.

Renal angiography

Renal angiography is the gold standard test for **renovascular disease**, but it is rarely used in this setting as there is little evidence that intervention alters prognosis. It can be useful in suspected **polyarteritis nodosa** where multiple aneurysms are visualised.

Dynamic nuclear medicine scans: MAG3 or DTPA

Mercaptoacetyltriglycine (MAG3) or diethylene triamine pentaacetic acid (DTPA) scans are both radio isotope scans using compounds labelled with 99m-technetium. The isotope is injected into the peripheral venous system and the compound is then taken up by the tubules and excreted through the renal system, which can be tracked using a gamma camera. It is useful to assess **split function** of each kidney (i.e. percentage contribution of each kidney to total function), **perfusion** and **obstruction**:
- If there is no perfusion, the kidney will not be visualised
- If there is obstruction the isotope will not pass beyond this level or there will be a delay if there is partial obstruction

Static nuclear medicine scan: dimercaptosuccinic acid

Radiolabelled dimercaptosuccinic acid (DMSA) scans are useful in the evaluation of renal scarring in **reflux nephropathy**. DMSA is given intravenously and then uptake is measured two to four hours later. Areas of scarring are visualized as areas of decreased uptake on the scan. This test can also assess split renal function.

Micturating cystourethrogram

A micturating cystourethrogram (MCUG) is used to detect **vesicoureteral reflux** by visualisation of the movement of radiocontrast in the urinary tract and bladder.

Histopathology

A renal biopsy is often required to make a definitive diagnosis, particularly when **glomerular disease** is suspected. Contraindications include:

- The presence of an uncorrectable bleeding diathesis
- Small kidneys
- A single functioning kidney
- Severe hypertension (>170/90 mm Hg)
- Active renal infection
- An uncooperative patient

A very large body habitus will make the procedure technically difficult.

Apart from establishing a diagnosis, biopsy can give additional information to guide further management. This includes staging of certain diseases (e.g. SLE) and the degree of active and chronic changes that may influence treatment and likelihood of response. For example, a large amount of chronic scarring detected in FSGS may deter initiation of high-dose steroids due to the small chance of recovery of renal function, compared with the risks of treatment.

2.4 Diagnostic approach

Diagnosis of kidney disease is often made following identification of abnormal kidney function on blood tests.

Acute kidney injury versus chronic kidney disease

One of the first considerations should be whether the kidney impairment is acute or chronic. By far the most reliable way to distinguish between the two is comparing current kidney function with historical values. Therefore, whether the patient is seen as an acute presentation or in an outpatient clinic, tracking down historical blood tests is invaluable to assess the rate of decline and is by far the most reliable method. Renal ultrasound may be helpful; small kidneys confirm CKD although there still may be an acute deterioration in kidney function superimposed on the chronic disease. Normal size kidneys can be seen in chronic kidney disease, particularly in people with diabetes.

Most blood parameters are not helpful in distinguishing acute from chronic kidney impairment. Complications such as anaemia and the calcium and phosphate abnormalities can develop over days. These abnormalities may also develop as part of the underlying aetiology, e.g. anaemia in microangiopathic haemolytic anaemia, low calcium in rhabdomyolysis. The only blood test that may have some value is the PTH concentration as a high concentration takes months to occur and indicates some degree of chronicity. Sometimes, when no previous blood tests are available and kidney size is normal, the degree of chronicity can only be evaluated on the renal biopsy.

If at all possible, urinalysis should be one of the initial tests performed. A bland urine, i.e. absence of significant blood and protein excludes most glomerular pathology. This significantly helps with the differential diagnosis of the underlying cause.

Complications of chronic kidney disease

If CKD is confirmed, evaluation of its complications (which include anaemia, bone mineral disease and vascular disease) should be undertaken (see Chapter 4). The underlying cause should also be considered, although sometimes a clear diagnosis is not possible when patients present with small kidneys and the renal acute screen is negative.

Cause of acute kidney injury

If AKI is confirmed, identification of the cause is important to ensure appropriate treatment and optimal chances of renal recovery. Whatever the underlying cause, there are some basic principles to follow, including:

- Optimisation of volume status and blood pressure
- Avoidance of nephrotoxic agents
- Appropriate dosing of renally excreted drugs

Gastric protection should also be considered and nutritional status should be addressed early.

If a patient presents with nephrotic syndrome, consideration should be given to the underlying pathology. In adults a renal biopsy is usually required. General supportive measures should also be undertaken and are discussed in Chapter 5.

2.5 Effects of drugs on the kidney

Many drugs can damage the kidneys. Some have predictable effects due to their mechanism of action or side effects, whereas others are idiosyncratic and unpredictable.

Common drugs causing predictable effects on the kidney

Non-steroidal anti-inflammatory drugs

NSAIDs most commonly affect the kidneys through haemodynamic compromise leading to acute injury. NSAIDs inhibit renal prostaglandin synthesis. In normal subjects, renal prostaglandins do not play a major role in regulation of renal haemodynamics. However, prostaglandin synthesis is increased by vasoconstrictors such as noradrenaline, vasopressin and angiotensin II. The latter is increased in effective volume depletion such as heart failure as well as salt and water losses. In these settings renal prostaglandins act to preserve renal blood flow and GFR by afferent arteriolar vasodilation. Inhibition of prostaglandin synthesis by NSAIDs can lead to afferent arteriole vasoconstriction and a decline in GFR. NSAIDs should therefore be avoided in those with renal disease or effective volume depletion.

Angiotensin-converting enzyme (ACE) inhibitors

Decline in GFR   A reduction in GFR is seen in some patients treated with ACE inhibitors, particularly those with chronic renal impairment, heart failure and bilateral renal artery stenosis. In these settings the intrarenal perfusion pressure is already reduced and maintenance of GFR is achieved by angiotensin-induced vasoconstriction, preferentially to the efferent arteriole.

Hence blocking this response with ACE inhibition will relax the efferent arteriole, lower intraglomerular pressure and reduce GFR.

When ACE inhibitors are started in patients at risk of this problem, such as those with suspected renal artery stenosis, renal function should be checked within one week of starting the drug. In some patients, there will be a modest increase in creatinine. However, a creatine rise or fall in estimated GFR of greater than 30% should prompt discontinuation of the ACE inhibitor. In most of these cases, renal function returns to baseline on cessation of the drug.

Hyperkalaemia   Angiotensin II along with high potassium concentrations increases the release of aldosterone, which is the major stimulus for urinary potassium excretion. ACE inhibitors block this effect and often cause a modest rise in potassium in patients with relatively normal renal function. However, more prominent hyperkalaemia may be seen in patients with renal insufficiency and cessation of the drug should be considered if potassium concentrations cannot be controlled.

Aminoglycosides
AKI resulting from aminoglycosides is due to ATN and is relatively common, affecting 10–20% of patients. The concentration of aminoglycosides in the proximal tubule cells can exceed the concurrent serum concentration, hence AKI can occur even with close monitoring.

Aminoglycosides should be avoided if at all possible in patients at risk of AKI. Strategies to minimise nephrotoxicity include reducing the dose, which may be down to 1 mg/kg using a once daily dosing regimen and limiting the duration of therapy to seven days. One dose of aminoglycosides may be sufficient until further microbiological information is available.

Iodinated contrast
Iodinated contrast media are used in angiography and CT. Their use can lead to AKI, which is often, but not always, reversible, and so should be avoided or used with caution in at-risk patients.

Contrast agents are believed to cause ATN by their vaso-constrictive effect as well as direct cytotoxic effects. Various iodinated agents have different levels of toxicity with the lowest risk with low-osmolar or iso-osmolar agents. Risk factors for contrast-induced ATN include:

- Underlying renal impairment
- Diabetic nephropathy
- Reduced renal perfusion (e.g. heart failure or hypovolaemia)
- High total dose of contrast agent

Typically a decline in kidney function occurs within 12–24 hours following contrast administration. Preventive measures are discussed in Chapter 3. The key strategy is proper hydration.

Gadolinium

Gadolinium is a non-tissue specific hyperosmolar contrast agent used in MRI. **Nephrogenic systemic fibrosis** is a fibros-ing disorder seen only in patients with renal impairment and associated with recent exposure to gadolinium. The risk of developing this condition following gadolinium exposure is estimated to be around 2.5–5%.

The initiating event is probably tissue deposition of gado-linium, resulting in marked fibrosis of the dermis. This leads to thickening of the skin overlying the extremities and trunk. Sys-temic involvement can include fibrosis of muscle and internal organs such as lungs causing reduced diffusion capacity; fibrosis of the diaphragm leading to respiratory failure; and pericardial fibrosis.

Clinical insight
Gadolinium should be avoided in all patients with a GFR <30 mL/min.

Idiosyncratic effect of some drugs
Nephrotic syndrome

Some drugs are associated with the development of minimal change disease or membranous nephropathy, which would both present as nephrotic syndrome. Known drugs include NSAIDs, associated with **minimal change disease**, and gold and penicillamine, which are associated with **membranous**

nephropathy. A history of use of these drugs should be sought in these settings.

Acute tubulointerstitial nephritis

Acute tubulointerstitial nephritis is most often caused by drugs, although there are other causes (see Chapter 10). Many drugs are associated with this condition, the most common being:

- NSAIDs
- Penicillins
- Allopurinol
- Proton pump inhibitors
- 5-aminosalicylates, e.g. mesalazine

Patients have an acute decline in kidney function accompanied by other clinical features such as rash (typically erythematous maculopapular over the trunk), fever, eosinophilia and white cell casts and white cells on urine microscopy. Management involves discontinuation of the drug and the possible use of corticosteroids.

Tubular disorders

Some drugs can cause proximal tubular dysfunction leading to what is called **Fanconi's syndrome**. This is when glucose, amino acids, bicarbonate and phosphate are passed into the urine rather than being reabsorbed by the proximal tubule. The antiretroviral drug tenofovir is a known cause, as are some chemotherapy agents.

2.6 Prescribing and renal impairment

Many drugs are excreted by the kidneys and require dose adjustment and closer monitoring in patients with renal impairment. It is advisable to check dosages in local renal prescription guidelines before prescribing.

Commonly prescribed drugs

More commonly prescribed drugs that require adjustment include antibiotics, opioids and heparin.

Antibiotics

Many antibiotics are renally excreted. Dose adjustment of individual agents should be checked and depends on renal function prior to administration.

Opioids

Absorption, metabolism and clearance of opioids are complex in renal impairment, where active metabolites of many of these drugs can accumulate. Codeine and morphine, for example, are not recommended as their active metabolites are particularly neurotoxic. If morphine is used, long-acting preparations should be avoided. Oxycodone, much of which is metabolised by the liver, and fentanyl, which is short acting, are safer but should still be used with caution and close monitoring.

Heparin

Low-molecular-weight heparins (LMWH) have a longer half-life in renal impairment and should be avoided in patients with a GFR of <20 mL/min. Unfractionated heparin should be used in this setting, which can be given subcutaneously as prophylaxis or intravenously as treatment for venous thromboembolism.

Prescribing in specific situations
End-stage kidney disease

In the context of end-stage disease, dose adjustment is required for renally excreted drugs. Consideration should also be given to removal of the drug by dialysis, which will vary depending on the type of dialysis. The timing of drug doses may therefore have to be adjusted. For example, gentamicin is mostly removed by haemodialysis and so should be given after, and not before, the procedure. Little gentamicin is removed by peritoneal dialysis and most removal is dependent on residual renal function.

> **Clinical insight**
>
> The major interaction to be aware of with azathioprine is allopurinol, which slows down elimination of the former. Therefore this combination should be avoided.

Kidney transplantation

In patients who are post-transplant, dose adjustment may be required for renally excreted drugs. Consideration should also be given to interactions with immunosuppressive agents. Commonly used agents to maintain immunosuppression are the calcineurin inhibitors ciclosporin or tacrolimus plus the anti-proliferative agents azathioprine, or mycophenolate mofetil. Calcineurin inhibitors are metabolised by the hepatic cytochrome P450 enzymes and so a variety of drugs that inhibit or induce this enzyme pathway can affect blood concentration.

Acute kidney injury

The kidneys are highly vascular organs: in order to maintain salt–water and acid–base balance, and excrete unwanted metabolites, they need to filter 1700 L of blood, and make 1–2 L of urine a day. The active and highly oxygen-dependent tubular cells are more exposed to toxins carried by the blood than any other cells in the body, and hence are very vulnerable to hypoxia and toxic injury. **Figure 3.1** shows a tubular cell with its brush border and numerous mitochondria.

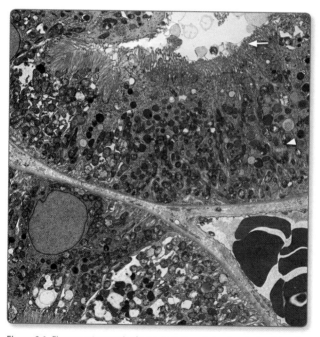

Figure 3.1 Electron micrograph of a renal tubular cell showing the brush border (arrow) and mitochondria (arrowhead). The numerous mitochondria in each cell utilise large quantities of oxygen for proper functioning of the tubular cell. By courtesy of Dr Ramzi Rajab, St George's Hospital, London.

Acute kidney injury (AKI) is a clinical condition diagnosed by a rise in creatinine and (usually) decreased urine output. The most common cause of this injury is damage to the tubular cells by hypoxia or toxins. Once damaged the tubular cells lose their architecture, such as the brush border, appear flat and take time to regenerate (see **Figure 3.2**). Other causes include immune-mediated glomerular or tubulointerstitial injury. Obstruction of the urinary tract is a less common cause, but promptly reversible; it should be considered and ruled out early in the diagnostic process.

3.1 Clinical scenarios

Chest pain, nausea and vomiting

Presentation

A 65-year-old man with type 2 diabetes was admitted with central retrosternal chest pain. He felt nauseous and had vomited a few

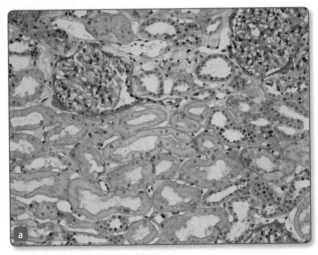

Figure 3.2 (a) Normal renal biopsy. (b, c) Haematoxylin and eosin section of a renal biopsy sample from a patient with acute tubular necrosis. Note the flattening of the tubular cells (b) with loss of the brush border, and debris in the tubular lumen consisting of damaged tubular cells (c). By courtesy of Dr Ramzi Rajab, St George's Hospital, London.

times prior to presentation. The electrocardiogram at presentation showed ST elevation myocardial infarction and his blood pressure was 116/70 mm Hg. He underwent a primary percutaneous

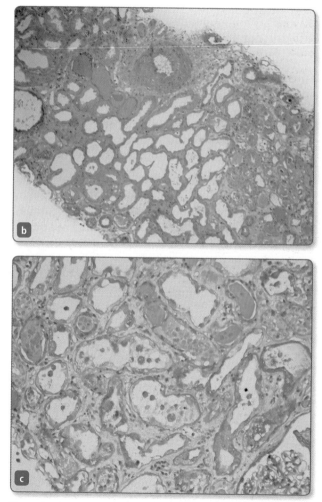

Figure 3.2 *Continued.*

coronary intervention during which his blood pressure was low. On the third day, his creatinine increases to 250 µmol/L from a baseline of 110 µmol/L and his urine output drops.

Diagnostic approach

The rise in creatinine and decreased urine output suggest a diagnosis of acute kidney injury. The possible causes could be radiocontrast injury or volume depletion. However, other causes such as obstructive uropathy need to be ruled out.

Further history

His regular medications prior to admission included losartan, aspirin, atorvastatin and insulin. On careful questioning, it is found that he had hardly any fluids on the day of his admission and had felt dry in his mouth. His systolic blood pressure remained <100 mmHg for about 6 hours during the coronary intervention.

Diagnostic approach

The low blood pressure could have caused decreased kidney perfusion, resulting in low oxygen levels in the kidney and tubular damage. He had taken losartan on the day of admission; this impairs the autoregulation of blood flow in the kidney, which would otherwise have maintained intraglomerular pressure in the face of a fall in systemic blood pressure by angiotensin-mediated efferent arteriolar vasoconstriction (**Figure 3.3**). Hence prerenal renal failure is a possible cause for the rise in his creatinine; radiocontrast injury is equally possible. Glomerular disease needs to be ruled out.

Further investigations

Urine examination shows no blood and a trace of protein; microscopy shows no dysmorphic red cells or casts. His urine sodium concentration is 60 mmol/L with an osmolality of 250 mOsmol/L. Renal ultrasound shows two 11 cm kidneys with no obstruction. His serum creatinine kinase is normal.

Diagnostic approach

A diagnosis of **acute kidney injury** due to acute tubular necrosis related to radiocontrast injury is made. Glomerular disease is ruled out by the lack of red cells, casts or any significant proteinuria. The high sodium concentration in the urine rules out prerenal renal failure; normal ultrasound rules out obstructive uropathy (i.e. postrenal).

Further management
The patient is treated with intravenous normal saline and losartan is stopped to improve his blood pressure and prevent further kidney damage.

From day 4 to 7, his urine output increases, and by day 10 his creatinine concentration is back to normal.

Drowsiness in an intravenous drug user
Presentation
A 37-year-old male intravenous drug user is brought to the emergency department at 3 am by a friend. He had been on the floor for several hours, drowsy, after taking intravenous heroin the night before. He is drowsy and has a blood pressure of 126/80 mm Hg. He has bruising over his left thigh and his serum creatinine is 256 µmol/L with a potassium of 7.1 mmol/L. The electrocardiogram (ECG) shows a sinus rhythm, normal axis and 'tall tented' T waves.

Diagnostic approach
The creatinine and potassium levels allow a diagnosis of AKI with hyperkalaemia. The cause of the injury is not clear.

Immediate management
The hyperkalaemia is treated with intravenous calcium and insulin-dextrose. In the first hour of admission, his urine output is minimal despite 2 L of intravenous normal saline administration. Serum potassium after 1 hour is 6.5 mmol/L. The patient is transferred to the intensive care unit for continuous dialysis. It is noted that he has pain and difficulty in moving his left leg.

Further investigations

The patient's urine is dark brown and his uric acid concentration is 691 mmol/L. The serum creatinine kinase concentration is 180,560 units/mL (normal 40–320). His urine is positive for myoglobin but only minimal protein. His urine has no dysmorphic red blood cells (RBCs) or red cell casts. Ultrasound examination of the kidneys is normal. Serum calcium is 2.12 mmol/L and serum phosphate is 2.4 mmol/L.

Diagnostic approach

Raised creatinine kinase, potassium and phosphate in the blood indicate muscle breakdown as a possible cause of AKI. A normal kidney ultrasound, lack of dysmorphic RBCs or casts rules out obstructive uropathy or glomerular disease as the cause of kidney injury. A diagnosis of severe AKI due to rhabdomyolysis is made.

Further management

Three days later, the patient is fully awake and is discharged from the intensive care unit. He is continued on intermittent haemodialysis in the renal ward.

4 weeks after his admission, his creatinine shows improvement without dialysis, and he is discharged from the renal ward. His kidney function completely recovered over a period of 6 weeks.

This case demonstrates how toxins can cause severe kidney failure but the tubular cells can regenerate and make a complete recovery.

3.2 Acute kidney injury

AKI is defined as a clinical condition with a rise of creatinine of 1.5 times from baseline, or a 26.4 μmol/L rise from baseline and/or with a decrease in urine output of less than 0.5 mL/kg/h for more than 6 hours. With rising creatinine and decreasing urine output, AKI is classified into stages 1–3 (**Table 3.1**).

	Creatinine	Urine output
Stage 1	Rise 1.5–1.9 fold from baseline or ≥26.4 µmol/L	<0.5 mL/kg/h for >6 hours
Stage 2	Rise 2–3-fold from baseline	<0.5 mL/kg/h for >12 hours
Stage 3	Rise >3-fold from baseline or ≥354 µmol/L	<0.3 mL/kg/h for >24 hours or anuria for 12 hours

Table 3.1 Stages of acute kidney injury.

Epidemiology

AKI is common in hospitalised patients, occurring in up to 13%. The incidence of AKI increases with age, and it has been rising over the last few decades, particularly in the elderly. This is probably related to the increasing age of the population as a whole, the associated comorbidities, and the polypharmacy often seen in hospitalised patients. It is also important to note recent improvements in diagnosis by assessing for minimal changes in creatinine levels and urine output, and their association with increased mortality and length of hospital stay.

Causes

The causes of AKI are traditionally defined as (**Table 3.2**):
- Prerenal
- Renal
- Postrenal

Prerenal   Prerenal causes (e.g. hypovolaemia due to vomiting or diarrhoea) result in decreased renal blood flow and impaired renal tissue oxygenation. The kidney tries to maintain glomerular filtration by maintaining the pressure within the glomerulus with afferent arteriolar vasodilation (prostaglandin mediated) and efferent arteriolar vasoconstriction (angiotensin II mediated) (see **Figure 3.3**). The kidney also tries to maintain blood volume by retaining salt and water; hence the urinary sodium concentration, at least initially, is low. However, if the insult

Prerenal	Intrinsic renal	Postrenal
Volume depletion	Acute tubular necrosis	Ureteric obstruction
Decreased effective volume	Acute interstitial nephritis	Urinary bladder outflow tract obstruction
Altered intrarenal haemodynamics: 1. NSAID-induced afferent arteriolar constriction 2. ACEi/ARB-induced efferent arteriolar dilation	Acute glomerulonephritis	
	Vascular (small and large vessel diseases)	

Table 3.2 Causes of renal failure. ACEI, angiotensin-converting enzyme inhibitor. ARB, angiotensin II receptor blocker. NSAID, non-steroidal anti-inflammatory drug.

continues and the tubules are damaged, they can no longer retain salt and water and the urinary sodium loss increases.

Renal   Intrinsic renal injury can be immune mediated or caused by nephrotoxins. Immune-mediated kidney injury can be either glomerular or tubulointerstitial, and urine dipstick and microscopic examination are extremely helpful for diagnosis in these cases. Nephrotoxins include drugs such as antibiotics (e.g. aminoglycosides), chemotherapeutic agents (e.g. cisplatin) and radiocontrast agents. Toxins may also be generated within the body due to haemolysis or rhabdomyolysis.

It is important to remember that drugs can also cause impaired autoregulation. For example, angiotensin-converting enzyme (ACE) inhibitors can impair the efferent arteriolar vasoconstriction and non-steroidal anti-inflammatory agents can impair the afferent arteriolar vasodilation, which are necessary during hypotension to maintain a normal glomerular filtration rate (GFR). Drugs such as ampicillin and rifampicin can also cause an allergic reaction with lymphocytes and eosinophils in the tubolointestitium, causing acute interstitial nephritis and AKI (see Chapter 10).

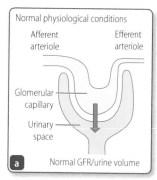

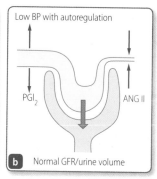

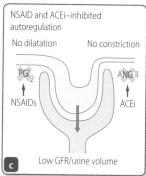

Figure 3.3 Effect of angiotensin-converting enzyme (ACE) inhibitors and non-steroidal anti inflammatory agents (NSAIDs) on normal renal autoregulation. (a) Normal physiological conditions. (b) Autoregulation in the presence of systemic hypotension: dilation of the afferent arteriole by PGI_2 and constriction of the efferent arteriole by angiotensin II to maintain GFR. (c) Interruption of autoregulation by ACE inhibitors and NSAIDs. BP, blood pressure. ANG, angiotensin. GFR, glomerular filtration rate. PGI2, prostaglandin I2. NSAID, nonsteroidal anti-inflammatory drug. ACEi, angiotensin-converting enzyme inhibitor.

Postrenal Obstructive uropathy causing AKI is seen in approximately 10% of patients. It is a rare cause in the intensive care unit, as AKI is usually due to factors other than obstruction and most patients have a urinary catheter, but the diagnosis is very important as the obstruction can be relieved once the diagnosis is made.

Clinical features

The presenting symptoms of AKI can be variable and often non-specific, such as nausea, tiredness or lethargy. A history of decreased urine output, if present, is useful. However, the different causes can sometimes be identified with a good history and examination as follows.

Prerenal injury   Patients can present with diarrhoea and vomiting coupled with dizziness and weakness indicating volume depletion and hypotension. Bleeding after a major trauma can cause hypotension and dizziness. A detailed fluid intake and output analysis sometimes reveals volume depletion as a cause when this is not obvious from the initial history. Physical assessment of volume status is essential for both diagnosis and management of AKI. Indicators of hypovolaemia are:

- Low blood pressure
- Postural hypotension
- Tachycardia
- Loss of skin turgor
- Dry mucous membranes

Drug-induced renal disease   A careful drug history is very important particularly for ACE inhibitors, angiotensin receptor blockers (ARBs), chemotherapeutic agents, aminoglycosides, penicillins and other antibiotics. Joint pains and maculopapular erythematous skin rash are features associated with allergic interstitial nephritis.

Vasculitis, autoimmune and other intrinsic renal disease

- A history of skin rash, palpable purpura, joint pains, blood in urine or smoky urine can indicate vasculitis as a cause of AKI
- Oral ulcers, loss of scalp hair and facial rash, particularly in a young woman, can be due to lupus nephritis
- A purpuric rash in a young person over the legs or buttocks is typical of Henoch–Schönlein purpura
- A history of muscle injury with dark urine could indicate rhabdomyolysis
- Jaundice and dark urine could be caused by haemolysis
- Sepsis is associated with fever, chills and rigors

Obstructive uropathy   A history of poor urine flow, hesitancy and precipitancy suggest obstructive uropathy. A careful examination of the abdomen is important to rule out a palpable urinary bladder. It is usually a smooth mass rising from the pelvis and dull to percussion. With pressure during palpation patients report an urge to pass urine.

Pathogenesis of acute tubular necrosis

Renal tubules are vulnerable to trauma by hypoxia and/or toxins such as contrast agents (see the first *clinical scenario* above) or toxins released after muscle trauma (see the second *clinical scenario* above).

> **Clinical insight**
>
> Occasionally, patients present late with AKI, and are volume overloaded, as evident from ankle swelling, raised jugular venous pressure, high blood pressure, a third heart sound, and lung crepitations. Volume overload that cannot be managed by diuretics may be an indication for dialysis.

Hypoxia (or the toxin) causes decreased adenosine triphosphate (ATP) production in the tubular cells, which in turn damages the actin cytoskeleton within the tubular cells. It also damages the adhesion molecules anchoring the tubular cells to the basement membrane and to each other. The tubular cells malfunction due to loss of polarity and, with persistent injury, they drop off into the tubular lumen and cause obstruction. In the early stages of mild tubular malfunction, the condition is reversible. In the late stages when tubular cells are damaged and drop off, the condition becomes irreversible (**Figure 3.4**). Recovery then involves a regeneration of tubular cells over a period of time, as with the patient with rhabdomyolysis in which it took several weeks for renal function to recover.

Investigations

The diagnosis of AKI is established by serum creatinine and urea measurement.

Urine dipsticks test   Urine examination with simple dipsticks can identify glomerular diseases causing AKI when there is the presence of significant proteinuria (usually 4+) and haematuria.

Urine biochemistry   Measurement of urinary sodium and osmolality is useful in distinguishing reversible prerenal renal failure and established acute tubular injury. A low urine sodium (<10 mEq/L) concentration with high urine osmolality establishes a diagnosis of prerenal renal failure.

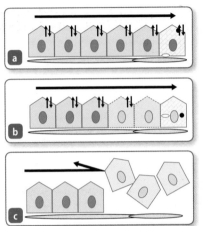

Figure 3.4 The pathogenesis of acute tubular necrosis, progressing from normal (a) to abnormal (b, c). (a) Normal tubular epithelial cells and normal urine flow are indicated by the long arrow from left to right. The tubular cell on the extreme right is cut open to demonstrate the actin cytoskeleton and tubular proteins, on the luminal side (black circle) and on the basement membrane (white oval). The peritubular capillary appears as a long thin gray tube under the tubular cells. (b) Reversible tubular damage, prerenal renal failure and some loss of polarity due to abnormal alignment of proteins. (c) Irreversible tubular damage with established acute tubular necrosis; dead tubular cells dropping off into the tubular lumen causing obstruction to urine flow.

Urine microscopy   This is useful to diagnose glomerular or interstitial injury as the presence of dysmorphic RBCs and red cell casts indicates glomerular disease whereas eosinophils and white blood cell casts indicate interstitial disease. Occasionally, crystals are identified in the urine indicating toxicity due to agents such as aciclovir and indinavir. It is important to use only freshly voided urine, and microscopic examination by an experienced person gives the best results.

Blood tests   Diagnosis of certain immune causes of AKI requires specific tests such as antinuclear antibody and complement for lupus nephritis, antineutrophil cytoplasmic antibody, antiglomerular basement membrane antibody, and serum electrophoresis and urine Bence Jones proteins for myeloma (see Chapter 6).

Ultrasound scanning   A kidney and bladder ultrasound scan is important to rule out obstructive uropathy.

Renal biopsy Occasionally, a renal biopsy may be required, particularly if there is a suggestion of glomerular disease which can be treated with immunosuppression; it is rarely needed if the clinical diagnosis is acute tubular necrosis.

Management

Early recognition and treatment of the causes of tubular injury such as toxins, drugs, hypovolaemia and sepsis can help aid recovery. Once the condition is diagnosed with a rise in creatinine or decrease in urine output, treatment should be implemented promptly.

Fluid resuscitation Replacement of fluids requires urgent attention. In the presence of hypovolaemia, fluid therapy using crystalloids should be started promptly. Colloids can be used in haemorrhagic shock. In cases where fluid therapy may be problematic, such as the presence of heart failure in association with AKI, small boluses of crystalloid are very useful, e.g. 250 mL of normal saline given rapidly, followed by careful examination for pulmonary congestion before the next bolus of fluid. If hypotension does not improve after 2 L of fluid resuscitation

Clinical insight

In prerenal renal failure, as the tubules are still functioning to some extent and the body is trying to conserve salt and water, the urinary sodium is low , usually <10 mEq/L. In established acute tubular necrosis, when the tubules are non-functioning, the urine cannot be concentrated and sodium is lost in the urine. Hence the urinary sodium is high, usually >20 mEq/L. If the urinary sodium results are equivocal, estimation of fractional excretion of sodium, which is defined as the ratio of urinary to plasma sodium/creatinine concentration, is useful (FeNa = urine sodium: plasma sodium/urine creatinine: plasma creatinine x 100). In prerenal renal failure, prior to the onset of acute tubular necrosis, the fractional excretion of sodium is less than 1%. This distinction is very useful as prerenal renal failure at this stage is reversible with fluid therapy.

Clinical insight

In bladder outflow tract obstruction, the urine bladder is enlarged, with thick walls and trabeculae if chronic. Chronic obstruction can be due to urethral valve or prostate hypertrophy. A unilateral hydroureter and dilated renal pelvis indicate the obstruction is at the vesicoureteric junction or above the level of the bladder. Ureteric obstruction may occur in the lumen, e.g. due to a renal stone, or caused by a condition outside the lumen, e.g. due to retroperitoneal fibrosis.

then senior (nephrology) review is required; further treatment may be best carried out in a high dependency unit setting. Once fluid resuscitation is complete, further replacement is guided by urine output; usually the requirement is for about 500 mL plus the daily urine output.

Antibiotics for sepsis   If the diagnosis of sepsis is made (increased white blood cell count, rise in C-reactive protein (CRP)), antibiotics should be started promptly.

Nephrotoxins   A careful review of the drug chart is important and agents such as ACE inhibitors, ARBs, and non-steroidal anti-inflammatory drugs should be stopped. If any drug is suspected of causing allergic interstitial nephritis (e.g. penicillins, rifampicin, proton pump inhibitors) it should be stopped. Certain drugs and antibiotics also require dose adjustments to prevent further kidney injury.

Intensive care management   Sicker patients with AKI and persistent hypotension, severe sepsis, hypoxia or drowsiness require management in the intensive care unit.

Dialysis   Dialysis is indicated in AKI in the presence of refractory hyperkalaemia, acidosis, volume overload or symptoms of uraemia. The use of diuretics in the prevention of AKI is not recommended. However, they may be useful if there is significant volume overload. The use of dopamine to prevent AKI is also not recommended.

Prevention

Contrast   Radiocontrast-induced AKI is common particularly during cardiac catheterisation. Proper hydration prior to contrast administration is the key in the prevention of AKI. The volume of contrast used should be minimised. An alternative investigation that does not require contrast administration may need to be considered. In the high risk patient, i.e. older people with diabetes and chronic kidney impairment, the patient should be admitted and given normal saline 1 mL/kg/h 12 hours before and 12 hours after to prevent radiocontrast nephropathy. A careful assessment of volume status during fluid resuscitation is necessary to avoid volume over load. *N*-acetylcysteine can be given (600 mg orally, twice a day) on the day before and on the day of contrast administration.

Postsurgical hypovolaemia   Volume depletion in postsurgical patients is also a common cause of AKI. Prompt recognition of hypovolaemia and its management in postsurgical patients is essential in the prevention of AKI.

Prognosis

AKI is potentially reversible, particularly when it occurs in isolation and there are few comorbid conditions. Mortality is uncommon, but is associated with increasing age and sicker patients. Overall, the presence of AKI in any hospitalised patient increases mortality and length of stay, with the adverse effects increasing with increasing peak serum creatinine concentration. A full or near full recovery is usual but some patients are left with chronic kidney disease, and occasionally the disease is end stage and patients become dialysis dependent for the rest of their life.

In summary, AKI is common in hospitalised patients and associated with high mortality; prompt diagnosis and management is the key to a better outcome. Sicker patients might require monitoring and management in the intensive care unit with the help of renal physicians, but most cases of mild to moderate AKI are reversible and can be managed by general physicians. Prevention of AKI by prompt removal of the causes of kidney injury such as nephrotoxic agents by all members of the team managing acutely unwell patients is very important.

Chronic kidney disease

In addition to excreting toxic waste products, the kidneys also maintain salt–water and acid–base balance, and function as an endocrine organ. In chronic kidney disease (CKD) all of these functions are impaired to a variable degree. CKD is a clinical condition caused by a variety of disease processes which lead to a sustained and irreversible reduction in glomerular filtration rate (GFR); this is often associated with hypertension, anaemia, mineral and bone disorders, and cardiovascular complications. CKD is divided into 5 stages according to the degree of reduction in GFR (**Table 4.1**).

4.1 Clinical scenario

Hypertension, tiredness and increasing serum creatinine

Presentation

A 65-year-old Caucasian woman with a history of hypertension was referred by her general practitioner for tiredness, lethargy and a gradual rise in her creatinine concentration from 150 μmol/L to 180 μmol/L over a period of three years.

Stage 1	GFR >90 mL/min/1.73 m^2 with haematuria/proteinuria
Stage 2	GFR 60–89 mL/min/1.73 m^2 with haematuria/proteinuria
Stage 3	GFR 30–59 mL/min/1.73 m^2
Stage 4	GFR 15–29 mL/min/1.73 m^2
Stage 5	GFR <15 mL/min/1.73 m^2 or on renal replacement therapy

Table 4.1 Stages of chronic kidney disease. The low estimated glomerular filtration rate (GFR), haematuria or proteinuria needs to be present for more than 3 months to diagnose chronic kidney disease.

Her blood pressure is 158/88 mm Hg; the rest of the physical examination is normal. She is taking amlodipine and simvastatin.

Diagnostic approach

The diagnosis of CKD is established by the persistently low estimated glomerular filtration rate (eGFR). In this patient, the eGFR has dropped from 32 mL/min per 1.73 m^2 to 26 mL/min per 1.73 m^2, representing a change from CKD stage 3 to the more advanced stage 4. It is helpful to obtain a renal ultrasound to confirm that there are no reversible factors.

Guiding principle

There are several formulae which can be used to estimate GFR, of which the most commonly used is the Modification of Diet in Renal Disease (MDRD) formula, which takes into account the patient's age, gender, ethnicity and creatinine concentration.

Further investigations

Further investigations show a haemoglobin of 10.5 g/dL (normochromic normocytic indices), calcium 2.3 mmol/L, phosphate 1.3 mmol/L, parathyroid hormone 7.5 pmol/L, cholesterol 3.8 mmol/L and low-density lipoprotein (LDL) cholesterol 2.1 mmol/L. On renal ultrasound, two small non-obstructed kidneys with increased echogenicity are seen; this latter feature is non-specific but often seen with CKD.

Diagnostic approach

The patient has a normochromic, normocytic anaemia; this is typical of renal anaemia. She also has a calcium concentration at the lower end of normal and an elevated phosphate concentration. This is due to the decreasing excretory and endocrine functions of the kidney (discussed later in the chapter). Future aspects of management will include:

- Control of blood pressure
- An attempt to improve quality of life
- Prevention of complications associated with CKD

4.2 Chronic kidney disease

CKD is diagnosed by a sustained reduction in eGFR to <60 mL/min/1.73 m² for at least three months, or persistent haematuria, proteinuria or structural abnormalities of the kidney.

Epidemiology

CKD is common, with a prevalence in the USA and Europe of 11–15%. The prevalence is higher in patients with hypertension, diabetes and in the elderly; prevalence may be increasing as all of these risk factors increase among the general population. In the UK, large studies from primary care have shown a prevalence of CKD stages 3–5 of about 5.5%.

The financial burden related to CKD is substantial. In the USA, 22% of the healthcare budget is spent on patients with CKD yet they constitute only 7% of the government-funded (Medicare) population.

Causes and pathogenesis

A number of disease processes are responsible for kidney damage that can result in end-stage disease. Most commonly, the initial insult is due to hypertension or diabetes. Once the initial insult is established, CKD tends to progress even in the absence of the initial insult (**Figure 4.1**). This is due to compensatory hypertrophy in the surviving nephrons once some of the neph-

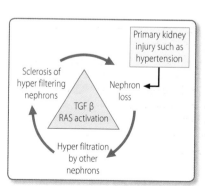

Figure 4.1 The progression of kidney injury. Activation of both RAS and TGF β are central to the mechanism of nephrosclerosis and ongoing damage.. RAS, renin–angiotensin system. TGF β, transforming growth factor β.

rons are injured. Hyperfiltration then causes further damage to groups of surviving nephrons, which become sclerosed and obsolete; in turn, further remaining nephrons undergo hyperfiltration and the process is perpetuated. Central to this ongoing damage is activation of the renin–angiotensin–aldosterone system (see **Figure 9.2**), and the effects of fibrotic cytokines such as transforming growth factor (TGF) β. In the chronically damaged kidney the glomeruli are sclerosed, tubules are atrophied and the interstitium is fibrosed (**Figure 4.2**).

Clinical features

CKD in the initial stages (mainly stages 1–3) is asymptomatic. Advanced kidney failure presents with non-specific symptoms, including tiredness, lethargy, loss of appetite, weight loss and nausea. Due to the kidney's lack of ability to concentrate urine, there is often increased nocturia and frequency; at lower levels of eGFR, salt and water retention tends to predominate. The underlying disease may also contribute to the symptoms, for example bone pains due to myeloma or abnormal vision due to diabetic retinopathy. The loss of the ability to maintain salt and water balance, acid–base balance, and endocrine dysfunction produces associated symptoms (**Table 4.2**).

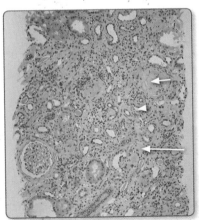

Figure 4.2 Histological picture of chronic kidney disease damage, showing glomerular sclerosis (arrow), tubular dropout (arrowhead) and interstitial fibrosis (long arrow). By courtesy of Dr Ramzi Rajab, St. George's Hospital, London.

Kidney abnormality	Altered mechanism	Effect	Management
Abnormal excretory function	Fluid retention	Hypertension	Salt restriction
	Potassium retention	Hyperkalaemia	Low potassium diet
	Phosphate retention	Hyperphosphataemia	Low phosphate diet
	Retention of acid	Metabolic acidosis	Sodium bicarbonate therapy
Lack of production of erythropoietin	Anaemia	Tiredness	Epoetin
		Left ventricular hypertrophy	Iron
Lack of production of 1,25 vitamin D	Hypocalcaemia	Bone pain	Vitamin D supplementation
	Increased parathyroid hormone	Fractures Osteomalacia Osteitis fibrosa	Phosphate-binders
Effect on cardiovascular health	Activation of RAAS	Left ventricular hypertrophy	ACEI, ARB
	Micro-inflammation	Coronary heart disease, CHF, arrhythmias	Blood pressure control <130/80 mmHg
	Hypertension		

Table 4.2 Abnormalities associated with chronic kidney disease, their manifestations and management. ACEi, angiotensin-converting enzyme inhibitor. ARB, angiotensin II receptor blocker. CHF, congestive heart failure RAAS, renin–angiotensin–aldosterone system.

Investigations

Once the diagnosis is established, investigations are focused on:
- Determining the aetiology
- Evaluating the complications related to CKD, such as anaemia, renal bone disease and cardiovascular complications

Urinalysis   Urine examination can be very helpful in determining aetiology. For example:

- Significant proteinuria of >1 g per day or a protein/creatinine ratio of >100 mg/mmol indicates glomerular disease. If seen in a (suspected) diabetic patient, together with other microvascular complications of diabetes such as retinopathy and neuropathy, this strongly suggests diabetic nephropathy
- Glomerular haematuria, i.e. dysmorphic red blood cells and red cell casts, suggests chronic glomerulonephritis
- Bence Jones proteinuria supports a diagnosis of myeloma, which may be suspected in an elderly patient presenting with renal impairment and hypercalcaemia

Ultrasound   An ultrasound scan of the kidneys is useful. It helps to rule out obstruction or cystic kidney disease as a cause of underlying kidney damage. It can also establish a diagnosis of CKD when the kidneys are smaller than normal and corticomedullary differentiation is lost, or the cortex appears irregular.

Renal anaemia   Anaemia in CKD is characteristically normochromic and normocytic; it is largely due to erythropoietin deficiency, which can be substituted with a variety of erythropoietin-stimulating agents. Before starting erythropoietin therapy, any deficiency of iron, vitamin B_{12} or folic acid should be corrected. With deficiencies of these essential nutrients, erythropoietin therapy is unlikely to work. It is also important that causes of ongoing red cell loss, such as gastrointestinal bleeding and haemolysis, or causes of chronic inflammation, which will lead to erythropoietin unresponsiveness, are excluded by clinical examination and relevant investigations.

Mineral and bone disorder in CKD

Mineral and bone disease in CKD is common and worsens as disease progresses. With advancing kidney damage there is decreased generation of 1,25 dihydroxy vitamin D, as the hydroxylation at the one position of the cholecalciferol molecule happens in the kidney. This lack of active vitamin D prevents absorption of calcium from the gut and hence the serum calcium concentration decreases.

The serum concentration of phosphate rises because of decreased renal excretion. Both low calcium and high phosphate increase production of parathyroid hormone. The elevated

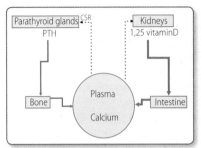

Figure 4.3 Mechanisms of calcium homeostasis. The calcium sensing receptor (CSR) on the parathyroid cells inhibits parathyroid production. Dotted lines indicate negative feedback. PTH, parathyroid hormone.

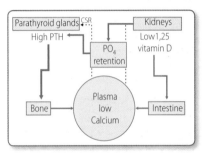

Figure 4.4 Abnormalities of calcium, phosphate, vitamin D and parathyroid hormone (PTH) in chronic kidney disease (see text for details). CSR, calcium-sensing receptor.

parathyroid hormone attempts to normalise the serum calcium by mobilising calcium from the bone (**Figures 4.3** and **4.4**). This combination of lack of active vitamin D (causing osteomalacia) and hyperparathyroidism (which causes bone resorption, resulting eventually in osteitis fibrosa), is termed renal osteodystrophy, and can cause bone pain and fractures.

Clinical insight

Cardiovascular complications of CKD

The risk of cardiovascular events in CKD patients is high, and increases as kidney function decreases. It is partly related to the presence of traditional risk factors such as diabetes and hypertension, which may of course be the underlying cause of the kidney disease. However, it also relates to the presence of certain non-traditional risk factors such as inflammation, anaemia, and mineral and bone disorders.

Management

The aims of CKD management are to:

- Prevent/delay disease progression
- Prevent/minimise the cardiovascular complications of kidney disease

- Treat anaemia
- Treat mineral and bone disorders
- Treat the underlying kidney disease if possible

In order to prevent both CKD progression and cardiovascular events, it is important to control both hypertension and diabetes. Blood pressure control will usually involve:

- Angiotensin-converting enzyme (ACE) inhibitors and/or angiotensin II receptor blockers (ARBs), as there is good evidence that use of these agents, particularly in patients with significant proteinuria, prevents progression of CKD
- Therapy with several antihypertensive agents
- Salt restriction – the importance of this cannot be over-emphasised

Diabetes management is based on good glycaemic control through lifestyle and dietary behaviours, as well as insulin therapy.

Anaemia   The treatment of CKD-related anaemia requires erythropoietin therapy, after essential hematinics (the chemicals required for eryth-ropoieses, including vitamin B12, folic acid and ferritin) have been replenished. Oral iron in advanced CKD is poorly absorbed, and in these patients intravenous iron therapy is useful.

> ## Clinical insight
>
> CKD is a common condition and the majority of the patients should be managed in the community by general practitioners. However, patients with progressive disease and/or associated complications will need referral to a nephrologist, particularly to plan renal replacement therapy.

Bone and mineral metabolism   The treatment of bone and mineral metabolism requires careful monitoring of calcium, phosphate and parathyroid hormone.

- In early CKD, when the parathyroid hormone tends to rise and 1,25-dihydroxyvitamin D concentrations are low, it is important to start the patient on 1,25-dihydroxy or 1-hydroxy vitamin D
- Later on as the phosphate levels continue to rise due to increased phosphate retention, dietary phosphate restriction is helpful, supplemented if necessary with a phosphate binder

Phosphate binders are available in either calcium containing or non-calcium containing forms; the non calcium containing phosphate binders have the possible advantage of helping to prevent vascular calcification. Phosphate binders should be taken with food so that they can bind the phosphate contained in food. After starting vitamin D and phosphate binders, patients need to be monitored to prevent hypercalcaemia and maintain phosphate concentrations at normal levels.

Prognosis

The majority of patients with well-controlled blood pressure have slow progression of their CKD. Most patients with CKD stages 1–3 will succumb to cardiovascular events, and few will progress to end-stage renal disease (ESRD) requiring dialysis therapy. Less than 1.5% of CKD stage 3 patients require dialysis over a period of five years, while 25% die of non-renal causes. However, certain kidney diseases such as diabetes or autosomal polycystic kidney disease may progress more rapidly. Such patients require proper education regarding the options for renal replacement therapy. They need advice on haemodialysis, haemodialysis access, peritoneal dialysis and kidney transplantation, the latter best done pre-emptively if possible, before dialysis becomes necessary.

4.3 End-stage renal disease

End-stage renal disease (ESRD) is a condition associated with symptomatic uraemia that requires renal replacement therapy for control of symptoms and survival. With decreasing kidney function, patients complain of increasing tiredness, lethargy, anorexia and nausea. These symptoms and fluid overload are indications for starting renal replacement therapy. Other biochemical indications can be hyperkalaemia, metabolic acidosis and very low eGFR, usually <10 mL/min/1.73 m^2. In 2009 in the UK the mean eGFR of patients starting renal replacement therapy was 9 mL/min/1.73 m^2.

Epidemiology

The incidence of ESRD in the UK was 109 per million in 2009. The majority of patients starting dialysis are middle aged or older with a mean age of 64.8 years. The prevalence of adult patients on renal replacement therapy was 49,000 at the end of 2009; 48% had kidney transplants, 44% were on haemodialysis and 8% on peritoneal dialysis.

The incidence of ESRD patients entering renal replacement therapy varies between countries. The incidence is high in the USA and Taiwan and very low in countries such as Bangladesh. It is partially related to the cost of renal replacement therapy. In the UK the cost of haemodialysis for one patient is approximately £34,000 a year.

Causes and pathogenesis

The most common causes of ESRD are diabetes, glomerulonephritis and hypertension. Of patients starting dialysis in the UK, 25% have ESRD from diabetes, 11% from chronic glomerulonephritis, 7% hypertension, and 6% have autosomal dominant polycystic kidney disease.

Clinical insight

Importance of predialysis care

Before starting renal replacement therapy, patients should be monitored closely in an advanced CKD clinic and have their treatment options clearly explained, so they can make an informed decision on which mode is best for them. Vascular or peritoneal access should be placed weeks or months before starting haemodialysis or peritoneal dialysis, respectively, so that the access is established at first use. An unplanned start of maintenance dialysis should be avoided as it results in poor outcome.

Clinical features

Most of the symptoms are very non-specific, comprising tiredness, lethargy, nausea, vomiting, anorexia and weight loss. Abnormal renal handling of salt and water can manifest as leg swelling, facial puffiness and even shortness of breath due to pulmonary oedema.

Investigations

Investigations regularly performed include renal function, bone profile, haematinics, hepatitis serology and parathyroid hormone measurements.

Regular monitoring for hepatitis C and human immunodeficiency virus (HIV) is important to prevent blood borne infection in haemodialysis units. Hepatitis B vaccination is essential for the same reason.

Management

Management of ESRD involves:

- Haemodialysis
- Peritoneal dialysis
- Transplantation
- Conservative approaches

Haemodialysis

Haemodialysis is the most common from of initial dialysis. In the UK in 2009, 70% of patients started renal replacement therapy with haemodialysis.

> ## Clinical insight
>
> Dialysis fluid is sterile and contains sodium, potassium, magnesium, calcium, glucose and bicarbonate. The concentration of potassium is lower and bicarbonate is higher in the dialysis fluid than the blood. This concentration gradient helps the patient to lose potassium and gain bicarbonate during dialysis. Waste products such as urea and creatinine are lost in the dialysis fluid moving from higher to lower concentration. The machine is also able to change the concentration of sodium, potassium and bicarbonate as necessary with each dialysis.

Method   Haemodialysis involves the use of a machine that pumps the patient's blood through an artificial filter three times a week, four hours at a time. This allows the transfer of waste products from blood to dialysis fluid, filtering across a semipermeable membrane.

Excess fluid is removed by applying a pressure gradient across the semi-permeable membrane. The machine can change the rate of fluid ultrafiltration by altering the trans-membrane pressure during dialysis. The process requires access to blood circulation via an arteriovenous fistula, arteriovenous graft (using a synthetic tube) or central venous catheter.

Complications   These include:

- Hypotension
- Bleeding
- Vascular access can clot and become unusable.
- Blood stream infection with Gram-positive organisms

Peritoneal dialysis

Peritoneal dialysis is less commonly used. It was used in 18% of incident dialysis patients in the UK in 2009.

Method   Peritoneal dialysis fluid, which is similar to haemodialysis fluid, is placed in the peritoneum using a catheter. Fluid is left in the peritoneum for a few hours for filtration to occur. The fluid, now containing waste products, is drained out and replaced with fresh dialysis fluid. This cycle is carried out by the patients 4 times a day while doing continuous ambulatory peritoneal dialysis. In automated peritoneal dialysis about 10 such cycles happen overnight. Patients need to be fit and capable of managing their own dialysis. The dialysis fluid contains a high glucose concentration to assist fluid removal via osmosis.

Complications   The main complication associated with peritoneal dialysis is infectious peritonitis. Good personal hygiene and meticulous asepsis while connecting the dialysis fluid bags to the catheter is necessary to prevent this. Hyperglycaemia, particularly in patients with diabetes, requires special attention as it can predispose to infections.

Kidney transplantation

Kidney transplantation is the ideal mode of renal replacement therapy, compared to long-term dialysis, as it improves quality of life and has the best long-term outcome. The main limitation is donor organ availability. The kidney donor can be live or dead. There is a long mean waiting time for receiving a cadaveric kidney in the UK (1110 days). Hence more and more patients are advised to receive a live donor kidney. In 2009 in the UK, about 2600 kidneys were transplanted with 38% from live donors.

Method   The recipient is assessed for both their suitability for major surgery, and their ability to tolerate immunosuppression and avoid post-transplant infection. After determination of the blood group and human leucocyte antigen (HLA) tissue type, the patient is placed on a nationwide waiting list. Patients are chosen from the list according to the matching of blood group and HLA type with the donor, as well as their age and amount of time they have been on dialysis. There is no waiting time if patients have their own related donor.

The donor kidney is placed in the iliac fossa and connected to both the external iliac artery and vein, and urinary bladder (**Figure 4.5**). All kidney transplant patients receive strong induction immunosuppression with intravenous corticosteroids and

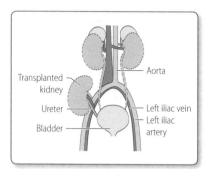

Figure 4.5 The position of a transplanted kidney.

interleukin-2 receptor antibody followed by oral calcineurin inhibitor (tacrolimus or ciclosporin), mycophenolate mofetil and tapering (i.e. gradually reducing dose) of corticosteroids.

Complications   The most common problems post-transplantation are rejection of the transplanted kidney, and infections with unusual organisms such as cytomegalovirus, *Pneumocystis jiroveci* and other fungi. In the long-term, malignancies, particularly of the skin and the lymphoproliferative system, are common. Hence, patients are followed up very closely in the post-transplant clinic.

Conservative

Some patients choose not to have renal replacement therapy due to comorbidities and poor quality of life which is unlikely to improve with dialysis. Patients who choose conservative management of their ESRD require ongoing care from their nephrologist and general practitioner for symptom control.

Prognosis

Prognosis of ESRD in dialysis patients is poor. Survival improves with kidney transplantation. The majority, up to one-half, of deaths are related to cardiovascular causes. In patients on haemodialysis, the annual mortality is approximately 20% with half of these being from cardiovascular causes. 6.5% of all deaths of haemodialysis patients are sudden cardiac deaths, which represents a high incidence.

Primary glomerular disease

Filter failure

The glomerulus is a filter (**Figure 5.1**): it lets some substances, such as water, electrolytes, and low-molecular-weight proteins through, while retaining others, including high-molecular-weight proteins and cells. Disease of the filter, whether primary (i.e. confined to the glomerulus) or secondary to a systemic illness, will cause retention of substances that should be freely filtered (i.e. a decrease in glomerular filtration rate (GFR)) and/or a loss of substances that should be retained (manifest as haematuria or proteinuria). Combinations of these two modes of filter failure, over various time courses, result in a small number of ways in which glomerular disease can present (**Table 5.1**).

Glomerular disease

Glomerular disease is usually seen as a difficult and confusing subject. There are three main sources of difficulty:

- With some exceptions, there is often no clear correlation between the presenting syndrome (see **Table 5.1**) and the

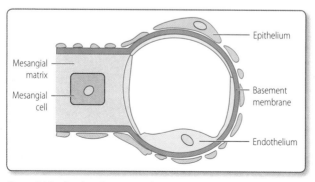

Figure 5.1 Capillary loop from a normal glomerulus.

Epithelium

Mesangial matrix

Mesangial cell

Basement membrane

Endothelium

Nephrotic syndrome	Heavy proteinuria (>3–5 g/day or equivalent)
	Hypoalbuminaemia (<30 g/L)
	Oedema
Asymptomatic urinary abnormalities	Haematuria and/or proteinuria
Nephritic syndrome	Haematuria, proteinuria and decreased glomerular filtration rate developing over a few days
Rapidly progressive glomerulonephritis	As for nephritic syndrome, but over weeks and months
Chronic kidney disease	Typically small kidneys with haematuria/proteinuria

Table 5.1 Presentations of glomerular disease.

underlying histopathological diagnosis (**Table 5.2**; this is why a renal biopsy is required for a confident diagnosis in most cases)
- The histopathological nomenclature is confusing, and varies between countries
- Again with some exceptions, the pathogenesis of many of the diseases is not understood

Although these difficulties cannot be avoided, the following approach can help minimise them:
- Consider primary glomerular diseases (the subject of this chapter, and the source of most of the conceptual difficulties) separately from secondary glomerular disease (Chapter 6)
- For the primary diseases, approach them under three separate domains:
  – Clinical presentation (see **Table 5.1**)
  – Histopathological diagnosis (see **Table 5.2**)
  – Pathogenesis (if known)

	Nephrotic syndrome	Asymptomatic urinary abnormalities	Nephritic syndrome	Rapidly progressive glomerulonephritis	Chronic kidney disease
Minimal change nephropathy	Usual				
Membranous nephropathy	Usual	Occasional			Occasional
Focal segmental glomerulosclerosis	Usual	Occasional			Occasional
IgA nephropathy	Rare	Usual	Rare	Rare	Occasional
Postinfectious glomerulonephritis	Rare		Usual		
Mesangiocapillary glomerulonephritis	Usual	Occasional	Occasional	Rare	Occasional

Table 5.2 How primary glomerular disease can present.

5.1 Clinical scenarios

Leg swelling

Presentation

A 55-year-old Caucasian man presents with progressive swelling of his legs. He first noticed this in his feet five weeks ago, but it has since extended to above his knees.

Diagnostic approach

Peripheral oedema is a common and often relatively non-specific finding, particularly in the elderly and patients on calcium channel blockers. Recent onset and significant progression should prompt consideration of more serious underlying disease (for example, of the heart, liver, or kidney).

Further history

There is no significant past medical history or allergies. The patient is on no regular medication. He does not smoke and consumes approximately 10 units of alcohol a week.

Examination

There is pitting oedema up to the mid thigh. No abnormalities are found on examination of the cardiovascular, respiratory or abdominal systems.

Diagnostic approach

The lack of other significant history or findings on examination should prompt consideration of a diagnosis of nephrotic syndrome. The urine should be tested; if there is no protein, nephrotic syndrome would be excluded.

Investigations

There is 4+ protein in the urine. Quantification gives a protein/creatinine ratio of 220 mg/mmol (normal <45). Nephrotic syndrome is confirmed by the finding of a low serum albumin concentration of 21 g/L (the normal range is 35–50).

Diagnostic approach

Following a diagnosis of nephrotic syndrome, the first step should be to consider possible secondary causes. In this case the absence of any other significant history or findings on examination makes a secondary cause, such as underlying neoplasm, diabetes, systemic lupus erythematosus (SLE) or amyloidosis unlikely.

- If any secondary cause of nephrotic syndrome is suspected, the relevant investigations should be ordered
- If a primary glomerular disease is suspected then, except in children, a renal biopsy is required to make a histopathological diagnosis

In this case, a renal biopsy is performed and shows membranous nephropathy.

> ### Clinical insight
>
> - In children, nephrotic syndrome is usually assumed to be caused by minimal change nephropathy, and treated as such without a biopsy
> - In adults, the primary causes are usually membranous nephropathy, minimal change nephropathy or focal segmental glomerulosclerosis; a biopsy is required to distinguish between these possibilities

Haematuria and proteinuria

Presentation

A 35-year-old man is found to have haematuria and proteinuria on dipstick testing during a routine insurance medical. He is also hypertensive with a blood pressure of 165/104 mmHg.

Diagnostic approach

Haematuria, if local causes and urinary tract infection have been excluded, should always be taken seriously as it can be the first presentation of renal tract malignancy. The initial assessment should attempt to determine whether a urological or nephrological referral is required.

Further history

The patient works in the finance industry. There is no significant past medical history and he is on no medication. He is a non-smoker.

Examination

Examination confirms raised blood pressure but is otherwise normal.

Diagnostic approach

In this case the patient's relative youth, absence of risk factors and presence of proteinuria and hypertension make a nephrological cause of the haematuria most likely.

> ## Clinical insight
>
> A complement profile is useful in the investigation of a suspected proliferative form of glomerulonephritis (presenting with nephritic syndrome, rapidly progressive glomerulonephritis, or asymptomatic haematuria with decreased eGFR) as hypocomplementaemia is seen in a relatively small number of conditions:
>
> - Postinfectious glomerulonephritis
> - Mesangiocapillary glomerulonephritis
> - Some immune complex mediated glomerulonephritides (e.g. SLE, infectious endocarditis, type II cryoglobulinaemia)

Investigations

Quantification of the proteinuria gives a protein/creatinine ratio of 55 mg/mmol. A full blood count is normal. Urea and electrolytes show a raised serum creatinine concentration of 136 µmol/L (normal range 60–110); this gives an estimated GFR (eGFR) of 52 mL/min. A complement profile and autoantibody screen are normal.

Diagnostic approach

The decreased eGFR confirms that this is most likely to be a nephrological problem. The normal complement profile is helpful in making a number of conditions less likely, but a renal biopsy is required for a definitive diagnosis.

A renal biopsy is performed, which shows immunoglobulin A (IgA) nephropathy.

5.2 Minimal change nephropathy

Minimal change nephropathy is so called because examination of a renal biopsy by light microscopy and immunohistochemistry is normal; the only changes are fusion of the podocyte foot processes seen on electron microscopy (**Figure 5.2**; compare with normal **Figure 5.1**).

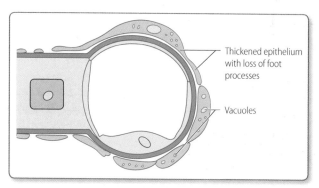

Thickened epithelium with loss of foot processes

Vacuoles

Figure 5.2 Capillary loop affected by minimal change nephropathy.

Epidemiology

This disease is the underlying diagnosis in over 75% of children presenting with nephrotic syndrome, and in approximately 30% of adult cases. Most cases are idiopathic, but there appears to be an association with allergy, and some cases occur in the context of malignancy, particularly Hodgkin's disease, and use of non-steroidal anti-inflammatory drugs.

Causes and pathogenesis

The cause is unknown. The associations described above, and the response to immunosuppression, suggest an immunological abnormality, but the details are obscure.

Clinical features

The presentation is uniform, with the vast majority of cases presenting with nephrotic syndrome (i.e. oedema); occasionally, patients will also notice frothy urine, particularly if it is a relapse and they are familiar with this symptom. Hypertension is sometimes found, particularly in adults.

Investigations

As always, secondary causes of nephrotic syndrome should be considered, and the appropriate investigations performed if indicated. The proteinuria should be quantified, and the eGFR estimated (this is usually normal, but may be decreased due to intrarenal oedema or hypovolaemia). The only abnormalities to be expected are a low serum albumin and raised cholesterol concentrations, common to all causes of nephrotic syndrome. In children, nephrotic syndrome is assumed to be due to minimal change disease and treated as such; a renal biopsy would only be performed if the nephrotic syndrome did not respond to treatment as expected. In adults a renal biopsy is required.

Management

The general principles of management of the nephrotic syndrome (whatever the cause) apply:

- Control of oedema with salt restriction and loop diuretics
- Control of hypertension with angiotensin-converting enzyme (ACE) inhibitors or angiotensin II receptor blockers, if present
- If possible, treatment of the underlying disease

Because of the hypercoagulability found in the nephrotic state, strong consideration should be given to anticoagulation if the serum albumin concentration is likely to be persistently lower than 20 g/L. This is not usually the case in minimal change nephropathy because of the rapid response to treatment.

Corticosteroids   Specific therapy consists of corticosteroids. The response is usually rapid, with resolution of oedema over days or a few weeks, though it may take a few months in adults. In patients unresponsive to corticosteroids, or who relapse frequently when the drug is reduced or withdrawn, more intensive immunosuppression with drugs such as cyclophosphamide or calcineurin inhibitors may be indicated.

Prognosis

The prognosis in terms of renal survival is excellent; if there is deterioration of eGFR, another diagnosis (usually focal segmental glomerulosclerosis) should be suspected. However, patients may continue to have relapses over many years and suffer from the side effects of corticosteroids.

5.3 Membranous nephropathy

Membranous nephropathy is so called because of the thickening of the glomerular basement membrane seen by light microscopy (**Figure 5.3**). Immunohistochemistry shows that this thickening is due to the deposition of IgG in a granular pattern; electron microscopy localises these deposits to the epithelial (i.e. outer) surface of the glomerular basement membrane, with spikes of basement membrane material protruding between the deposits.

Epidemiology

This disease is the commonest primary glomerular cause of nephrotic syndrome in Caucasian adults. Most cases are idiopathic, but up to 10% may be associated with underlying malignancy, usually carcinoma, and occasionally with certain drugs and infections (notably hepatitis B).

Causes and pathogenesis

Membranous nephropathy occurring in the setting of malignancy or infection is probably due to the deposition of immune complexes containing tumour or microbial antigens. Until recently, the target of the IgG in the deposits in idiopathic membranous nephropathy was unknown; recent evidence

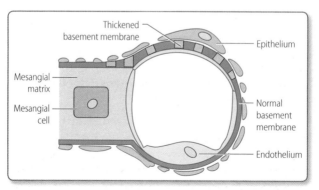

Figure 5.3 Capillary loop from a glomerulus with membranous nephropathy.

suggests that in many cases this may be the phospholipase A_2 receptor.

Clinical features

Presentation is with nephrotic syndrome, or on occasion, lesser degrees of proteinuria found on dipstick testing. Hypertension and renal impairment may also be found.

Investigations

Secondary causes of nephrotic syndrome, and the possibility of underlying infection or malignancy, should be considered and investigated as appropriate. Proteinuria should be quantified, and the eGFR estimated. A renal biopsy is required for a definitive diagnosis.

Management and prognosis

The nephrotic state should be managed as described for minimal change nephropathy. The prognosis of this disease is usually given in thirds:

- A third will go into a spontaneous remission
- A third will have persisting heavy proteinuria but preserved eGFR
- A third will experience persisting proteinuria and a deteriorating eGFR

Usual practice is to reserve additional treatment for patients with persisting nephrotic range proteinuria and/or deteriorating eGFR. For these patients immunosuppression with ciclosporin A, or a combination of corticosteroids and cytotoxic agents (known as the Ponticelli regimen), may be considered.

5.4 Focal segmental glomerulosclerosis

Focal segmental glomerulosclerosis is characterised by areas of sclerosis, mesangial matrix expansion, and collapse of capillary loops affecting, at least initially, only parts (segmental) of some glomeruli (focal) (**Figure 5.4**).

Epidemiology

This is the commonest primary glomerular cause of nephrotic syndrome in Afro-Caribbean adults. The majority of cases

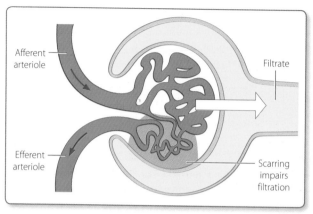

Figure 5.4 A glomerulus with focal segmental glomerulosclerosis. Part of this glomerulus is affected by a segmental lesion. Other glomeruli may be normal or globally sclerosed (the disease process is focal).

are idiopathic, but some occur in the setting of obesity, hyperfiltration in the presence of a reduced nephron mass, malignancy, and a number of other miscellaneous conditions.

Causes and pathogenesis

This condition is not a single entity, but represents a common pattern of glomerular injury produced by a number of different insults. Some rare cases, particularly in children, are due to genetic defects in a variety of podocyte proteins. Some cases are associated with the presence of a circulating proteinuric factor; this subgroup is particularly prone to recurrence in a transplanted kidney. In most cases the cause is unknown.

Clinical features

Presentation is often with nephrotic syndrome, but lesser degrees of proteinuria, hypertension and renal impairment are common.

Investigations

Proteinuria should be quantified and the eGFR estimated. Possible secondary causes should be investigated if indicated. A renal biopsy is required for definitive diagnosis.

Management and prognosis

The nephrotic state should be managed as described for minimal change nephropathy. The prognosis of this condition is poor, with up to two thirds of cases experiencing progressive deterioration of eGFR. Additional treatment is usually reserved for patients with persisting heavy proteinuria and/or decreasing eGFR, and here high-dose corticosteroids or other immunosuppressants may be considered.

5.5 IgA nephropathy

The disease is characterised by an increase in mesangial matrix and cells, in association with mesangial deposition of IgA (**Figure 5.5**).

Epidemiology

This is the commonest primary form of glomerulonephritis in the world, being found in up to 25% of renal biopsy series. The vast majority of cases are primary, but some may occur in the setting of liver disease and spondyloarthropathies.

Causes and pathogenesis

The cause is unknown. One current theory is that there is an abnormality of glycosylation of IgA.

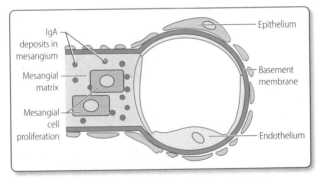

Figure 5.5 A capillary loop from a glomerulus with IgA nephropathy.

Clinical features

Presentation is usually with asymptomatic urinary abnormalities; a subset of patients have recurrent visible haematuria in association with infections (particularly respiratory infections). Presentations with nephritic syndrome, nephrotic syndrome or a rapidly progressive glomerulonephritis are rare. Hypertension is common.

Investigations

Apart from variable degrees of proteinuria and renal impairment, investigations are usually unremarkable; 50% will have raised IgA concentrations. Typical cases without significant proteinuria or renal impairment can be managed presumptively without a renal biopsy.

Management and prognosis

The general principles of good blood pressure control with ACE inhibitors or angiotensin II receptor blockers apply. Approximately 20% of cases will experience progressive renal impairment, and further treatment is usually reserved for this population; there is no consensus but various forms of immunosuppression may be tried.

5.6 Postinfectious glomerulonephritis

Classically seen following a group A streptococcal infection, this pattern of glomerular injury exhibits proliferation, with an increase in mesangial and endothelial cells as well as infiltration by polymorphonuclear leucocytes. Characteristically there are hump-shaped subepithelial immune deposits (**Figure 5.6**).

Epidemiology

Poststreptococcal glomerulonephritis is still an important condition in some communities (e.g. indigenous population in Australia); in western Europe the condition is now seen more frequently as a sequela of other infections.

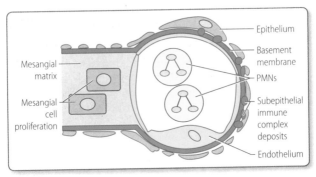

Figure 5.6 A capillary loop from a glomerulus with postinfectious glomerulonephritis. PMN, polymorphonuclear cell.

Causes and pathogenesis

The accepted mechanism is that of a planted antigen: circulating microbial antigens deposit in the glomerulus during the acute infection, and then serve as the target for an immune attack as the primary response develops one to two weeks after the infection.

Clinical features

Typically, presentation is an abrupt onset of nephritic syndrome two to three weeks after the inciting infection. Patients may have oedema and hypertension.

Investigations

As well as routine blood tests, a complement profile should be obtained as this is one of the conditions associated with hypocomplementaemia. There may also be evidence of the precipitating infection. Typical cases may be managed without a renal biopsy.

Management and prognosis

Patients with postinfective glomerulonephritis are managed with supportive care. Dialysis may be required in severe cases. Recovery usually occurs spontaneously, and the long-term prognosis is good, although occasionally progressive renal impairment is seen, particularly in adults.

5.7 Mesangiocapillary glomerulonephritis

This condition is characterised by an increase in mesangial matrix and cells, and thickening of capillary loops due to peripheral extension of mesangial cells and matrix, with the latter causing apparent double contouring of the basement membrane (**Figure 5.7**). Two main types (I and II) are recognised. In the USA the condition is more commonly termed membranoproliferative glomerulonephritis.

Epidemiology, causes and pathogenesis

The condition is found in around 10% of cases of nephrotic syndrome.

Type I   This is probably an immune complex disease, and in some cases this is due to a recognised underlying condition (lupus, infectious endocarditis, cryoglobulinaemia in association with hepatitis C infection); most cases are idiopathic

Type II   This is much rarer, and associated both with partial lipodystrophy and a circulating antibody that activates complement (C3 nephritic factor). There is evidence that this antibody causes both the renal disease and the lipodystrophy

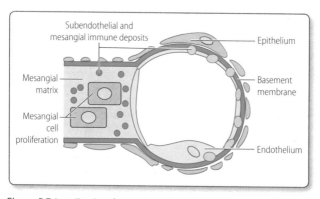

Figure 5.7 A capillary loop from a glomerulus with mesangiocapillary glomerulonephritis (type I).

Clinical features

Presentation is usually with nephrotic syndrome, but asymptomatic urinary abnormalities and a rapidly progressive glomerulonephritis may also be seen. Features of the underlying conditions mentioned above may be present.

Investigations

In addition to quantification of proteinuria and eGFR, a complement profile should be obtained, as this is one of the forms of glomerulonephritis characterised by hypocomplementaemia. Particular consideration should be given to investigating for lupus and hepatitis C. A renal biopsy is required for diagnosis.

Management and prognosis

In the absence of a treatable underlying disease the prognosis is poor, with most cases experiencing progressive renal impairment (particularly in the case of type II). There is some uncontrolled evidence suggesting that corticosteroids and other immunosuppressants may be helpful in some cases.

Secondary glomerular disease

As with the primary glomerular diseases considered in Chapter 5, the renal presentation of systemic disease involving the glomerulus is relatively stereotyped (**Table 5.1**); the difference is that the disease process usually involves other organ systems as well. However, this is not always the case. For example, antiglomerular basement membrane disease and small vessel vasculitis can be confined to the kidney. This can make the distinction between primary and secondary glomerular disease somewhat arbitrary, but it is still useful conceptually.

6.1 Clinical scenario

Skin rash

Presentation

A 75-year-old woman presents with a two-week history of a rash over her lower legs. Examination shows a palpable purpuric rash; there are a few splinter haemorrhages in her nails.

Diagnostic approach

A palpable purpuric rash indicates vasculitis, which is supported by the presence of splinter haemorrhages. Cutaneous vasculitis is often relatively benign, but its presence should prompt a search for more systemic features.

Further history

Further questioning reveals that the patient has been unwell for the last two to three months, with progressive malaise and decrease in appetite; she has lost 5–6 kg in weight. She has also noted some aches and pains in her wrists and knees over this period. There is no other significant history; she is on no medication.

Examination
Further examination reveals some tenderness of the wrist and knee joints. Dipstick testing of her urine shows protein 2+, blood 3+.

Clinical insight
The presence of palpable purpura, indicating vasculitis, together with systemic abnormalities plus or minus abnormalities in the urine should prompt urgent referral for further diagnostic investigations – this is a medical emergency.

Diagnostic approach
The malaise, weight loss and arthralgias, together with the presence of blood and protein in the urine, strongly suggest the diagnosis of a disease process such as systemic vasculitis.

Investigations
Blood tests show a normochromic normocytic anaemia (haemoglobin 10.3 g/dL, normal range 12–16), significant renal impairment (serum creatinine concentration of 382 μmol/L, normal range 60–110) and a positive antineutrophil cytoplasmic antibody with a perinuclear staining pattern (perinuclear antineutrophil cytoplasmic antibodies; p-ANCA). Further testing shows that the p-ANCA pattern is due to the presence of antimyeloperoxidase antibodies.

Clinical insight
It is important to establish the time course of deterioration in renal function in new patients with renal impairment because whether the deterioration has occurred over years or a shorter time frame will make a considerable difference to the differential diagnosis, and the urgency with which investigations should be pursued.

Diagnostic approach
In any patient presenting with unexpected renal impairment, it is important to try to establish the time course of deterioration in renal function. In this case, the patient had an incidental blood test performed four months previously, which showed a normal serum creatinine concentration. This pattern of deterioration of renal function over a small number of weeks or months, together with blood and protein in the urine, is very typical of rapidly progressive glomerulonephritis (see **Table 5.1**).

In the appropriate clinical setting – which rapidly progressive glomerulonephritis certainly is – the presence of a positive p-ANCA and myeloperoxidase (MPO) antibodies, or similarly a combination of cytoplasmic antineutrophil cytoplasmic antibodies (c-ANCA) and antiproteinase 3 antibodies, is very specific and sensitive for the diagnosis of a small vessel vasculitis.

Given the potential seriousness of the diagnosis, and the consequent treatment, histological confirmation is helpful. A renal biopsy is therefore carried out, which shows a focal necrotising glomerulonephritis with crescent formation (i.e. a proliferation of cells in Bowman's space; see **Figure 6.1**).

6.2 Vasculitis

Vasculitis is inflammation of blood vessels. This may be primary (the subject of this section) or secondary to another disease process, such as the connective tissue diseases considered in the next section. Of the primary disorders, the most important are the small-vessel necrotising vasculitides associated with ANCA positivity, which are the main focus of this section.

Other primary vasculitides that can involve the kidney include Henoch–Schönlein purpura and macroscopic polyarteritis nodosa.

- Henoch–Schönlein purpura consists of a purpuric rash, arthralgia, abdominal pain and renal involvement; renal biopsy shows changes very similar to those found in IgA nephropathy (see Chapter 5), usually with crescentic change
- Macroscopic polyarteritis nodosa, if defined strictly as only involving large or medium-sized blood vessels, is very rare; renal biopsy shows ischaemic changes only, as there is no glomerular involvement (the glomerulus is a modified small blood vessel). Neither of these diseases is characteristically ANCA-positive

Epidemiology, causes and pathogenesis

ANCA-positive vasculitis can affect any age but occurs more commonly in older age groups. At least in part due to the wider availability of ANCA assays, these diseases are being recognised

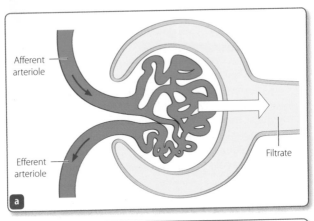

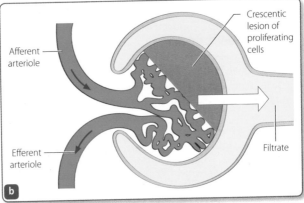

Figure 6.1 (a) A normal glomerulus. (b) A glomerulus with a focal necrotising crescentic lesion (arrow).

more frequently, with incidence rates in the range of 10–20 per million per year.

The cause of ANCA-positive vasculitis is unknown. There are some weak epidemiological links to exposure to silica, and individual cases may be precipitated by infections or certain drugs (e.g. propylthiouracil).

Clinical features

A number of different patterns may be seen:

- Granulomatosis with polyangiitis (Wegener granulomatosis) classically involves the kidney, upper and lower airways with a granulomatous pattern of inflammation
- Microscopic polyangiitis, in which most organ systems can be involved
- Renal-limited vasculitis
- Churg–Strauss syndrome is a distinct entity characterised by allergy (usually asthma), vasculitis and eosinophilia

The renal presentation of all of these is usually as a rapidly progressive glomerulonephritis, with other features depending on the precise pattern of organ involvement. Lung involvement, causing pulmonary haemorrhage, is sometimes seen, giving a clinical picture very similar to antiglomerular basement membrane disease (see Section 6.4).

Investigations

The key investigations are an ANCA blood test and a renal biopsy.

ANCA Most cases of active, primary small-vessel vasculitis will be ANCA-positive, but a negative result does not exclude the diagnosis.

Renal biopsy This usually shows a focal necrotising glomerulonephritis with crescent formation (see **Figure 6.1**); staining for immunoglobulin deposits is negative, or minimally positive, in contrast to other causes of crescentic nephritis considered in Sections 6.3 and 6.4.

Management

Treatment involves immunosuppression, with corticosteroids and cyclophosphamide used for induction; rituximab may be an alternative to cyclophosphamide in selected cases. Whether plasma exchange is a useful addition to induction is at present unclear. Maintenance treatment is with corticosteroids and azathioprine.

Prognosis

The prognosis has improved with current treatment regimens, with even dialysis-dependent patients likely to recover independent renal function. Continued follow-up is mandatory, as up to a third of patients will experience a relapse.

6.3 Systemic lupus erythematosus and other connective tissue diseases

A number of connective tissue diseases can involve the kidney, but the most important is systemic lupus erythamatosus (SLE), the main focus of this section. Rheumatoid arthritis may involve the glomerulus with secondary amyloidosis (considered below in Section 6.6), drug toxicity, or as part of a vasculitic flare. The renal crisis seen in systemic sclerosis involves intrarenal arterioles, with a pattern of 'onion skinning' very similar to that seen in accelerated hypertension (see Section 9.4).

Epidemiology

SLE is a common disease, with a prevalence of 1 in 2000–3000 women, rising to approximately 1 in 200–300 in African American women. Renal involvement is also common, being present on simple clinical criteria (proteinuria, urine sediment, renal function) in up to two thirds of patients at diagnosis. More severe forms of involvement are rarer, but make a significant contribution to morbidity and mortality when present.

Causes and pathogenesis

The main contribution to renal pathology in SLE (lupus nephritis) is via the deposition of immune complexes. Depending on the amount and properties of these complexes a number of different patterns are seen, ranging from relatively trivial involvement, through more aggressive proliferative forms (including crescent formation), to a pattern similar to idiopathic membranous nephropathy, and more chronic, scarring variants.

Clinical features

These reflect the diversity of the pathology: lupus nephritis can present with any of the patterns of glomerular disease set out in **Table 5.1**. Combinations of the various presentations may occur within an individual, either simultaneously or at different stages in the course of the disease.

Investigations

In addition to quantification of proteinuria and glomerular filtration rate (GFR), key tests are the relevant autoantibodies (e.g. antinuclear or anti-double-stranded DNA antibodies), a complement profile and a renal biopsy.

Management

A renal biopsy is useful in guiding treatment, as more aggressive immunosuppression is only indicated for the more severe proliferative patterns, and sometimes the membranous variant. In these cases treatment has traditionally been induction with corticosteroids and cyclophosphamide, followed by maintenance with corticosteroids and azathioprine. Recent evidence suggests that mycophenolate mofetil is equivalent to cyclophosphamide for induction, and superior to azathioprine for maintenance.

Prognosis

Treatment has considerably improved the outlook in the more severe forms of lupus nephritis. However, the outlook is variable, and close monitoring of patients is indicated.

6.4 Antiglomerular basement membrane disease

Antiglomerular basement membrane disease is also known as Goodpasture disease. Strictly, the original description was of pulmonary haemorrhage and glomerulonephritis (i.e. 'Goodpasture syndrome'), a presentation probably seen more often with small vessel vasculitis (Section 6.2).

Epidemiology

This devastating disease is rare, with an incidence of 1–2 per million per year.

Causes and pathogenesis

The disease is due to the presence of an autoantibody which

binds to collagen components present in the alveolar and glomerular basement membranes.

Clinical features

Presentation is with rapidly progressive glomerulonephritis. Pulmonary haemorrhage is not always seen: it is commoner in smokers, or those with some other cause of lung injury. Even when present, pulmonary haemorrhage may be largely concealed, with little overt haemoptysis.

Investigations

The key investigations are a blood test for antiglomerular basement antibody (a screen for ANCA is also done because of the overlap in clinical presentation) and a renal biopsy. Biopsy shows a necrotising crescentic glomerulonephritis, distinguished from other causes by the presence of linear staining for immunoglobulin along the basement membrane. Lung haemorrhage may be suggested by transient air space shadowing on the chest X-ray, and/or a raised carbon monoxide transfer factor (T_LCO).

Management and prognosis

Treatment is immunosuppression (as for small-vessel vasculitis) with the addition of plasma exchange to remove the antibody. If the patient presents on dialysis, there is less than a 10% chance of recovery of independent renal function; in such cases aggressive treatment may be reserved for those with pulmonary haemorrhage.

6.5 Diabetic nephropathy

The kidney is one of the many target organs affected by the complications seen in long-standing diabetes mellitus, both types I and II. It is unusual to have significant diabetic nephropathy without evidence of microvascular disease in other organs (e.g. diabetic retinopathy).

Epidemiology

Owing to the high (and increasing) prevalence of type 2 diabetes, diabetic nephropathy accounts for about a third of the patients on end-stage renal failure programmes in Western societies. In type 1 diabetes, in which the time of onset is usually well defined, the median time to the development of overt diabetic nephropathy is about 15 years. There is some evidence that the incidence of nephropathy is dropping in more recent cohorts, perhaps as the result of improvements in glycaemic and blood pressure control.

Causes and pathogenesis

Changes to the glomerular basement membrane and other structures result in glomerulosclerosis. Occasionally this occurs in a nodular pattern (Kimmelstiel–Wilson lesion, **Figure 6.2**).

Clinical features

During the development of diabetic nephropathy there is usually a progression of proteinuria from normal through to microalbuminuria (i.e. increased protein excretion but below the threshold detected by dipsticks) to overt proteinuria, which may be in the nephrotic range. During this evolution the GFR, although raised initially, progressively falls towards end-stage renal failure.

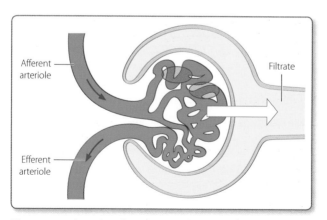

Figure 6.2 A glomerulus affected by diabetic nephropathy and showing a nodular sclerosing pattern (Kimmelstiel–Wilson lesion).

Investigations

Quantification of proteinuria by measuring the albumin/creatinine ratio plays an important role in the monitoring of diabetic patients. Unusual features (absence of microvascular disease elsewhere, haematuria) may suggest the need for a renal biopsy, as other coincidental glomerular pathology is always possible.

Management and prognosis

The cornerstones of management are good glycaemic and blood pressure control. Recommended targets for blood pressure are <140/80 mmHg (or <130/80 mmHg if there is kidney, eye or cerebrovascular disease). Angiotensin-converting enzyme (ACE) inhibitors or angiotensin II receptor blockers are the favoured choice of drug in most patients.

Patients with end-stage renal disease due to diabetes tend to do poorly, largely due to vascular complications in other territories. However, selected patients may still benefit from renal transplantation or, in younger patients with type 1 diabetes, kidney-pancreas transplantation.

6.6 Myeloma

A number of conditions are due to the deposition of paraproteins in the kidneys. These are monoclonal immunoglobulins or parts of immunoglobulins produced by an underlying B cell or plasma cell clone which may or may not be malignant. Myeloma is probably the commonest of these disorders, and renal impairment is a not uncommon presentation of myeloma.

Pathogenesis and clinical features

The pattern of immunoglobulin deposition usually seen is tubular rather than glomerular, producing the characteristic 'myeloma kidney' seen on biopsy: tubular casts which fracture and produce an inflammatory response. Under these circumstances there may be renal impairment but little in the way of proteinuria, as Bence Jones protein (immunoglobulin light chains produced by malignant B cells) is not detected by protein dipsticks.

Light chains may also deposit in the glomerulus as amyloid (primary amyloid light-chain (AL) type) or, in a different ultrastructural form, as light chain deposition disease. These patterns are usually associated with significant proteinuria, which may be in the nephrotic range. A similar picture is seen as a complication of the amyloid deposited in some cases of chronic inflammation (the serum amyloid A protein, giving AA type amyloid).

> **Clinical insight**
>
> In elderly patients presenting with significant renal impairment but no proteinuria, think of two conditions in particular: renovascular disease (see Chapter 9) and myeloma. Suspect myeloma particularly in the presence of hypercalcaemia.

Investigations

Investigations include serum electrophoresis, skeletal survey (an X-ray series of the whole body), and examination of the bone marrow. A renal biopsy may also be indicated if there is doubt about the diagnosis.

Management and prognosis

Treatment is directed at the myeloma itself, which will usually determine the prognosis. Hypercalcaemia, if present, should be corrected. Plasma exchange to remove circulating paraprotein is controversial.

6.7 Cryoglobulinaemia

Several conditions are characterised by the production of immunoglobulins that have the physicochemical property of precipitating in the cold, the commonest and most important of which is type II (mixed) cryoglobulinaemia.

Causes and pathogenesis

Type II cryoglobulinaemia is due to the production by an abnormal B cell clone of a monoclonal rheumatoid factor, usually of IgM class. Because it is a rheumatoid factor, the IgM will bind polyclonal IgG, producing large amounts of circulating immune complexes containing both IgM and IgG (i.e. mixed).

These complexes can deposit in various organ systems, such as skin, joints, kidney, and viscera. After deposition, they activate complement via the classical pathway, and set up an inflammatory response. In many cases the abnormal B cell clone is associated with infection by the hepatitis C virus.

Clinical features

Arthralgias, a purpuric skin rash and hepatomegaly are the commonest extrarenal manifestations. Renal involvement may produce asymptomatic urinary abnormalities, nephritic syndrome, nephrotic syndrome, or a rapidly progressive glomerulonephritis.

Investigations

Skin biopsy will show a leucocytoclastic vasculitis. Renal biopsy usually shows a type I mesangiocapillary glomerulonephritis (see Chapter 5). Serology will show high concentrations of rheumatoid factor and evidence of marked activation of complement via the classical pathway. Evidence of an underlying hepatitis C infection should be sought.

Management

Any underlying disease such as hepatitis C should be treated. Acute exacerbations may be managed with high-dose corticosteroids, other forms of immunosuppression and plasma exchange.

Prognosis

The outlook is good if an underlying condition can be treated; in other cases the outcome is variable, with some patients progressing to end-stage renal failure.

6.8 Thrombotic microangiopathies

These conditions are characterized by endothelial injury and the deposition of thrombi in the microcirculation, including the glomeruli. The fibrin strands in the microcirculation cause shear damage to the red blood cells, producing the schistocytes and microangiopathic haemolytic anaemia (MAHA) typical of the conditions. The two main entities are:

- Haemolytic–uraemic syndrome (HUS) – MAHA plus renal failure
- Thrombotic thrombocytopenic purpura (TTP) – MAHA, renal failure, thrombocytopenia, central nervous system involvement and pyrexia.

Causes and pathogenesis

Haemolytic–uraemic syndrome   HUS may be congenital (due to deficiencies in certain of the control proteins of the alternative complement pathway) or acquired. The most important acquired form is seen following infection with verotoxin-producing *Escherichia coli*, which may be on an epidemic scale.

Thrombotic thrombocytopenic purpura   TTP may also be congenital due to a deficiency of an enzyme (ADAMTS13) that cleaves large-molecular-weight forms of von Willebrand factor. More commonly the same picture is due to acquired autoantibodies to the same enzyme.

Other conditions   Finally, a group of miscellaneous conditions may exhibit variable features of HUS or TTP depending on the extent of organ involvement. These diverse causes of endothelial damage include infections, malignancy, drugs (notably calcineurin inhibitors), pregnancy, accelerated hypertension and autoimmunity (such as the antiphospholipid syndrome).

Clinical features

These take the form of the features outlined above, plus those of any underlying predisposing condition. The renal picture is usually one of acute kidney injury. Nervous system involvement in TTP usually takes the form of an encephalopathy. The conditions may fluctuate in severity on a day-to-day basis. The congenital forms of both TTP and HUS tend to be recurrent.

Investigations

Investigations are directed towards target organ involvement. Regular monitoring of platelet count and lactate dehydrogenase (LDH) concentration as markers of disease activity is helpful.

Management

General care is supportive, with renal replacement therapy if indicated; any underlying condition should be treated if possible.

Haemolytic–uraemic syndrome For HUS due to verotoxin – antibiotics should be avoided; any other treatment is controversial. For HUS due to deficiencies of complement control proteins – treatment is difficult; control of complement activation with monoclonal antibodies is possible but extremely expensive.

Thrombotic thrombocytopenic purpura For TTP – plasma exchange with the appropriate replacement fluid (thereby both removing an autoantibody, if present, and replacing the missing enzyme) is indicated.

Electrolyte disorders

Maintenance of concentrations of the electrolytes in plasma is essential for homeostasis. Tonicity of plasma is maintained within a narrow range to avoid osmotically driven movement of water into or out of cells leading to cell growth or shrinkage with consequent damage.

Most potassium in the body is inside cells and most sodium is in the extracellular compartment. Maintenance of the potassium gradient across cell membranes is critical to the electrical potential difference across the cell membrane that is required for the generation of action potentials. Regulation

Guiding principle

When interpreting results for electrolyte concentrations in plasma, remember that a high or low concentration does not necessarily reflect a high or low total body content of the electrolyte. This is particularly true for sodium, where abnormalities in plasma sodium concentration are more often due to loss or retention of water than loss or retention of sodium.

of plasma calcium concentration is also important for appropriate generation of action potentials.

7.1 Clinical scenarios

Hyponatraemia

Presentation

A 24-year-old man sustained a head injury in a motorcycle accident and is currently on the intensive care unit. His serum sodium concentration has fallen from 140 mmol/L on admission 5 days ago to 124 mmol/L.

Diagnostic approach

Hyponatraemia is either due to the inability to excrete water or from loss of sodium.

Further history

He has not been treated with drugs known to cause hyponatraemia and has not drunk excessive volumes of water or been infused with large volumes of 5% glucose. There has been no vomiting or diarrhoea.

Examination

Physical examination indicates that he is euvolaemic.

Investigations

Lab tests show:
- Serum potassium is 4.3 mmol/L
- Urinary sodium concentration is 100 mmol/L
- Plasma osmolality is 270 mosmol/kg
- Urine osmolality is 800 mosmol/kg
- Cortisol and thyroid blood tests are normal

Diagnostic approach

Syndrome of inappropriate secretion of antidiuretic hormone (vasopressin) (SIADH) is a recognised complication of head injury. In this case, endocrine causes were excluded by normal cortisol and thyroid blood tests. Low plasma osmolality with high urine osmolality and normal urinary sodium concentration in a euvolaemic patient suggests water retention due to vasopressin excess in the absence of other potential causative factors.

Hyperkalaemia

Presentation

A 67-year-old Caucasian man with a 10 year history of type 2 diabetes mellitus was recently noted to have positive proteinuria on dipstick testing, a blood pressure of 160/94 mm Hg and serum creatinine concentration of 148 μmol/L. Treatment with ramipril was started and when he attended for follow-up one week later, his serum potassium concentration was 7.2 mmol/L.

Diagnostic approach

Potassium can be artefactually elevated in blood samples that have taken a long time to arrive in the laboratory even in the absence of obvious haemolysis. Haemolysis and a very high white blood cell or platelet count can also cause pseudohyperkalaemia. A serum potassium of greater than 6.5 mmol/L is a medical emergency, requiring immediate management pending results of a confirmatory blood test.

Further history

Apart from ramipril (an angiotensin-converting enzyme (ACE) inhibitor), he is taking no other medication that is known to either contain potassium, or block renal potassium excretion. Having been diagnosed as hypertensive, the patient uses a salt substitute based on potassium chloride in an attempt to reduce his sodium intake. A dietary history also reveals a diet rich in high-potassium foods.

Examination

Blood pressure is 144/88 mmHg with a heart rate of 72/min. The patient is euvolaemic.

Diagnostic approach

The hyperkalaemia here is likely to be due to ramipril blocking the renin–angiotensin system, leading to reduced aldosterone secretion with reduced elimination of potassium in an individual who has renal impairment. He is at risk of hyporeninaemic hypoaldosteronism due to diabetic nephropathy, which may also contribute to acidosis, leading to movement of potassium out of cells into plasma. He has a high dietary potassium intake.

Investigations

An electrocardiogram (ECG) shows typical hyperkalaemic changes (**Figure 7.1**; see also **Table 7.3** later in the chapter). Serum creatinine is 160 μmol/L, sodium is 142 mmol/L and bicarbonate is 18 mmol/L. Full blood count is normal.

Diagnostic approach

The rise in serum creatinine of around 10% indicating a fall in glomerular filtration rate (GFR) is typical on starting ACE inhibition and probably has only a minor role in the patient's

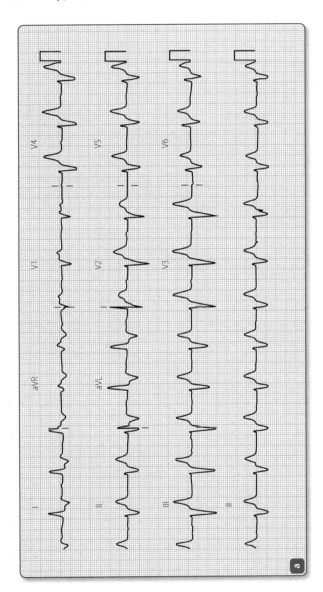

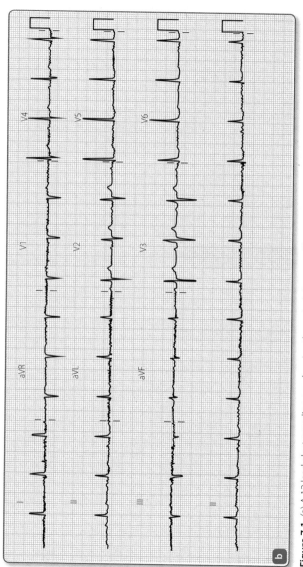

Figure 7.1 (a) A 12 lead electrocardiogram showing the typical changes of hyperkalaemia – prolonged PR interval, prolonged QRS complex, with tented T-waves. The ECG was taken when the patient's serum K+ concentration was 7.4 mmol/L. (b) An ECG from the same patient following haemodialysis to return serum K+ to the normal range with resolution of the ECG abnormalities.

hyperkalaemia. The low venous bicarbonate suggests metabolic acidosis. Normal plasma sodium makes primary mineralocorticoid deficiency unlikely.

7.2 Hyponatraemia

The conventional definition of hyponatraemia is a plasma sodium concentration <135 mmol/L but clinical consequences are uncommon until plasma sodium falls below 125 mmol/L, or falls rapidly (>20 mmol/L in 24 hours).

Causes

Hyponatraemia is caused by water retention, sodium loss or a combination of the two. A key point to remember is that plasma sodium concentration does not equate to total body sodium content, and it is more common for hyponatraemia to be due to retention of water diluting the plasma sodium than to be due to sodium loss. Causes of hyponatraemia are summarised in **Table 7.1**.

> **Guiding principle**
>
> For both hyponatraemia and hypernatraemia it is more common for abnormalities in water intake or excretion to be responsible, than primary problems with sodium retention or loss.

Pathogenesis

SIADH is due either to dysregulated or constant release of vasopressin from the posterior pituitary or to resetting of the osmostat with release of vasopressin at inappropriately low plasma osmolality. Sodium wasting is usually due to failure to reabsorb sodium in the renal tubule either through inherited or acquired defects in tubular cell function or mineralocorticoid deficiency. Water normally comprises 93% of plasma, the remainder is proteins and lipids. Hyperproteinaemia or hyperlipidaemia can reduce the water fraction to 80% leading to underestimation of the sodium concentration in the aqueous phase: pseudohyponatraemia.

Clinical features

Hyponatraemia is usually asymptomatic unless there has been a rapid fall in plasma Na^+ resulting in neurological complications

Excessive intake or retention of water	Vasopressin (ADH) release in response to hypovolaemia, nausea or pain
	Syndrome of inappropriate ADH secretion (SIADH):
	• Malignant disease: small cell lung cancer, thymoma, lymphoma, sarcoma, mesothelioma, pancreatic carcinoma
	• Pulmonary disease: pneumonia, tuberculosis, empyema
	• Neurological: head injury, infection, neoplasm, intracranial bleeding
	Drugs: MDMA (Ecstasy), antidepressants, carbamazepine
	Primary polydipsia
	and spondyloarthropathies.
	Water irrigation with glycine or sorbitol after transurethral prostatectomy (TURP)
	Congestive cardiac failure
	Cirrhosis
	Advanced renal failure
	Conditions associated with hypoalbuminaemia
	Hypothyroidism
	Pregnancy
Renal sodium loss	Diuretic treatment
	Mineralocorticoid deficiency
	Tubular disorders
Other sources of sodium loss	Vomiting
	Diarrhoea
Pseudohyponatraemia	Hyperproteinaemia
	Hyperlipidaemia

Table 7.1 Causes of hyponatraemia.

due to cerebral oedema caused by osmotic pressure driving water into cells. Symptoms include:

- Nausea
- Headache
- Fatigue, lethargy
- Muscle cramps
- Confusion
- Obtundation with seizures
- Coma and respiratory arrest in severe cases

With chronic hyponatraemia, cells lose osmolytes over a period of several days, removing the tendency for the cells to swell. However, this does lead to problems with excessively rapid correction of hyponatraemia when water is drawn out of cells by osmosis leading to shrinkage.

Approach to the patient

Look for clinical evidence of potential causes of SIADH, including cardiac failure, chronic liver disease or hypothyroidism. Management is guided by clinical assessment of intravascular volume to determine whether the patient is:

- Fluid-overloaded
- Euvolaemic
- Volume deplete

Investigations

Key investigations are:

- Serum creatinine and electrolytes
- Blood glucose
- Urinary sodium concentration
- Osmolality of plasma and urine

Hyponatraemia is usually associated with hypo-osmolality (plasma osmolality <275 mOsmol/kg). The combination of hyponatraemia and normal or elevated plasma osmolality indicates the presence of an additional, osmotically active substance (e.g. glucose, mannitol, urea in advanced chronic renal failure or ethanol).

Management

For hyponatraemia with plasma osmolality >275 mosmol/kg, management should be directed at the underlying condition. When plasma osmolality is <275 mosmol/kg, intravascular volume status should guide management, aiming to raise plasma Na^+ by no more than 8 mmol/L in 24 hours to avoid neurological complications including central pontine myelinolysis.

Hypovolaemic hyponatraemia In this situation diuretics should be discontinued and antiemetics administered if required. Intravascular volume should be restored by intravenous infusion of 0.9% NaCl. The amount of sodium required to achieve the desired plasma sodium can be calculated as follows:

$$Na^+ \text{ requirement (mmol)} = 0.6 \times \text{body weight in kg} \times (\text{desired } Na^+ - \text{actual } Na^+)$$

The volume of 0.9% saline (150 mmol/L) to be given over 24 hours can be calculated from this formula.

Euvolaemic hyponatraemia In this condition:
- Diuretics should be discontinued and the patient treated for hypothyroidism or mineralocorticoid deficiency
- Water intake should be restricted to 1 L/day
- Demeclocycline should be considered if there is no response to fluid restriction

Hypervolaemic hyponatraemia In this condition, water intake should be restricted to 1 L/day. Sodium intake should be restricted as total body sodium may actually be elevated and eating salt drives thirst. Diuretic treatment and potassium replacement may be required.

Euvolaemic or hypervolaemic hyponatraemia Patients can be treated with a vasopressin receptor antagonist to promote water diuresis without loss of sodium.

Neurological complications Hypertonic saline should be reserved for patients with seizures or other life-threatening neurological complications of hyponatraemia, given under expert supervision in a closely monitored environment.

Prognosis and complications
Hyponatraemia is an independent risk factor for mortality in hospitalised patients. The main complications are neurological.

7.3 Hypernatraemia

Hypernatraemia is serum sodium concentration >145 mmol/L, but is usually only clinically significant if the concentration is >155 mmol/L, or there has been a rapid rise (>20 mmol/L in 24 hours).

Causes and pathogenesis

Hypernatraemia is almost always due to water loss with inadequate replacement rather than to sodium gain. In patients who have access to water, increased plasma tonicity due to ingestion of sodium usually leads to thirst and drinking dilutes the plasma sodium into the normal range.

Inability to access water or inadequate drinking due to blunted thirst mechanisms with ageing are the commonest causes of hypernatraemia. Diabetes insipidus, either due to impaired vasopressin secretion (central) or nephrogenic due to failure to respond to vasopressin by mobilising aquaporin in the walls of the collecting ducts prevents appropriate reabsorption of water. Therapeutic diuretics and osmotic diuresis due to hyperglycaemia can lead to disproportionate loss of water. Sodium gain can be caused by the ingestion of sea water or infusion of large volumes of 8.4% sodium bicarbonate.

Clinical features

The symptoms of hypernatraemia range from mild confusion to coma.

Approach to the patient

Identify restricted access to, or excessive loss of, water, as well as sources of excess sodium. Assess intravascular volume as patients are often hypovolaemic in addition to being dehydrated.

Investigations

Check serum creatinine and electrolytes and blood glucose.

Management

The first step should be to stop water loss, which may involve giving an antiemetic, stopping diuretics or treating diarrhoea. Water deficit can be calculated from the equation:

$$H_2O \text{ deficit (L)} = \text{body weight in kg} \times 0.6 \times [(\text{actual Na}^+(\text{mmol/L}) - 140)/140]$$

Aim to replace one third of the water deficit per 24 hours in addition to replacing ongoing fluid losses and maintenance requirements. In a patient who is able to drink the safest way to replace water is by mouth, or if they cannot drink, nasogastric water administration should be considered. If intravenous replacement is required, 5% glucose equates to giving water. Check serum Na^+ daily: it should not fall by >8 mmol/L per 24 hours.

Prognosis and complications

As with hyponatraemia, the main complications of hyper-natraemia are neurological.

> **Clinical insight**
>
> Calculation of the water deficit is an essential step in the management of the hypernatraemic patient. It is usually greater than would be expected intuitively.

7.4 Hypokalaemia

The normal plasma potassium concentration is tightly regulated within the range 3.5–4.7 mmol/L.

Causes

In most cases hypokalaemia is due to excessive renal loss either due to drugs inhibiting tubular re-uptake of potassium, endocrine factors or inherited tubular defects (**Table 7.2**). The commonest cause of hypokalaemia is diuretic treatment, more so with thiazides but also with loop diuretics that increase sodium delivery to the distal nephron and promote the exchange of sodium for potassium.

Use of non-prescribed diuretics or laxatives for weight control should be considered in patients with unexplained hypoka-laemia. Ingestion of large amounts of liquorice can mimic the effects of mineralocorticoid excess. Processes driving potassium into cells, e.g. acute alkalosis, can cause hypokalaemia without a change in total body K^+. In the absence of a physiological abnormality, dietary potassium deficiency is extremely rare as the kidney is able to stop eliminating potassium.

Excessive renal loss	Drugs • Diuretics acting before the distal convoluted tubule (thiazides, loop diuretics, osmotic diuresis) • Carbonic anhydrase inhibitors • Penicillin and analogues (carbenicillin) • Renal tubular toxins (amphotericin B, aminoglycosides, cisplatinum, foscarnet) Endocrine • Primary mineralocorticoid excess: Conn syndrome, Cushing disease or ectopic adrenocorticotropic hormone (ACTH) secretion, glucocorticoid-remediable hyperaldosteronism • Secondary mineralocorticoid excess: renovascular disease, cardiac failure, hepatic failure • Functional mineralocorticoid excess: 11β-hydroxylase or 17α-hydroxylase deficiency, liquorice ingestion Defects in renal tubular function • Recovery from acute tubular necrosis • Bartter syndrome • Gittelman syndrome • Liddle syndrome Bicarbonaturia • Distal renal tubular acidosis (type I) • Treatment of proximal renal tubular acidosis (type II) • Chronic alkalosis Magnesium deficiency
Gastrointestinal losses	Diarrhoea (especially secretory) Laxative abuse Ureterosigmoidostomy
Shift of extracellular potassium into cells	Acute alkalosis (including persistent vomiting) Insulin treatment (patients with diabetic ketoacidosis are usually hyperkalaemic at presentation and become hypokalaemic after treatment with insulin) Vitamin B_{12} treatment β-adrenergic agonists Barium ingestion Theophylline, caffeine Familial hypokalaemic periodic paralysis Thyrotoxicosis
Inadequate dietary intake (unusual)	

Table 7.2 Causes of hypokalaemia.

Pathogenesis

The gradient of potassium concentration across the cell membrane is part of the mechanism that maintains the electrical potential across the cell membrane which is critical to the generation of action potentials. Minor changes in the plasma potassium concentration can significantly alter the resting membrane potential with impact on the excitable tissues: nerves and muscles, including cardiac muscle.

Clinical features

The majority of patients with hypokalaemia are asymptomatic. Symptoms can include generalised muscle weakness (rarely leading to paralysis or rhabdomyolysis), fatigue, constipation or paralytic ileus and pseudo-obstruction. Ascending paralysis may occur with serum K^+ <2 mmol/L. The main concern in hypokalaemic patients is the propensity to cardiac arrhythmias, primarily tachyarrhythmias, particularly in patients with pre-existing cardiac disease. Symptoms are more likely when there has been a rapid change in the plasma potassium concentration. Typical ECG changes are summarised in **Table 7.3**.

Approach to the patient

History should establish whether the patient has been vomiting or taking drugs predisposing to hypokalaemia. Blood pressure should also be checked.

Investigations

Check serum creatinine and electrolytes, magnesium, blood glucose and the ECG. Urinary potassium can help to confirm excessive urinary losses.

Guiding principle

Hypokalaemia tends to lead to tachyarrhythmias while hyperkalaemia prolongs intervals on the ECG, ultimately leading to asystole or ventricular fibrillation.

Management

Potassium supplements should be given to any patient with a serum potassium concentration <3 mmol/L, or <3.5 mmol/L if they are taking a drug where arrhythmic side effects

Electrolyte abnormality	ECG changes	Arrhythmias
Hypokalaemia	ST segment depression, flat T waves, U wave, extrasystoles	Atrial fibrillation, supraventricular tachycardia, ventricular tachycardia including torsades de pointes
Hyperkalaemia	Peaked T waves with progression to loss of T wave with severe hyperkalaemia, prolonged PR interval, wide QRS, shortened QT interval	Asystole, ventricular fibrillation
Hypocalcaemia	Prolonged QT interval	Ventricular fibrillation, heart block
Hypercalcaemia	Shortened QT interval	Uncommon

Table 7.3 Electrocardiographic (ECG) changes with electrolyte abnormalities.

are enhanced by low potassium or who have cardiac disease. Supplements should be given with caution in patients with renal impairment.

A plasma K^+ of 3 mmol/L secondary to potassium loss represents a total deficit of around 200 mmol (2 mmol/L – 600 mmol). Oral replacement is preferable – it is certainly safest. The usual dose is 40–120 mmol/day.

Intravenous replacement should be reserved for those with symptoms, or with K^+ <2 mmol/L or intolerant of oral potassium replacement. Infuse potassium into a large peripheral vein or central venous cannula at up to 20 mmol K^+/h (not more than 200 mmol/day).

If plasma K^+ is <2 mmol/L with arrhythmia, 80–100 mmol K^+ may be given over one hour.

Clinical insight

Remember that the risks of iatrogenic hyperkalaemia are potentially more serious than those of hypokalaemia.

Prognosis and complications

With treatment the risk resolves. The most dangerous

complication is the risk of tachyarrhythmias which may proceed to cardiac arrest.

7.5 Hyperkalaemia

While hyperkalaemia is strictly a plasma K^+ >4.7 mmol/L, it is unusual for there to be problems with K^+ <6.0 mmol/L.

Causes

Hyperkalaemia arises with reduced renal excretion or with a shift of potassium from the intracellular to the extracellular compartment. Table 7.4 summarises the causes of hyperkalaemia.

Pathogenesis

Potassium and hydrogen ions are exchanged across most cell membranes and secretion of one in the distal nephron tends to result in retention of the other. There is a tendency for potassium to diffuse passively out of cells down its concentration gradient that is countered, primarily, by a sodium/potassium ATPase. Hyperkalaemia reduces the resting membrane potential of the cardiac myocyte with subsequent decrease in the cardiac myocyte conduction velocity.

Clinical features

The most important clinical problem is cardiac arrhythmias, in particular, asystole and ventricular fibrillation. The most extreme ECG manifestation (Table 7.3) is the loss of the P wave with widening of the QRS complex to mask the T wave, producing the so-called sine-wave ECG (Figure 7.1). Hyperkalaemia can also cause weakness of skeletal muscle.

Approach to the patient

Check for sources of potassium intake and potassium-retaining drugs. Look for clinical signs of corticosteroid deficiency (i.e. Addison disease).

Investigations

Serum creatinine, full blood count, plasma glucose, arterial pH and plasma bicarbonate concentrations, and plasma cortisol if indicated, should be measured. An ECG should be taken.

Reduced renal excretion	Release of potassium from cells
Reduced glomerular filtration rate (acute or chronic renal failure)	Acidosis
Diuretics acting on the distal nephron (potassium-sparing), e.g. amiloride	Artefact due to potassium moving out of cells in a blood sample with delay in analysis
High-dose trimethoprim (amiloride-like action)	Cell lysis (tumour lysis syndrome, rhabdomyolysis, haemolysis, trauma, burns)
Drugs inhibiting the renin–angiotensin system (β-blockers, direct renin inhibitors, angiotensin-converting enzyme inhibitors, angiotensin II receptor blockers, spironolactone)	Insulin deficiency
Mineralocorticoid deficiency (Addison disease, hyporeninaemic hypoaldosteronism: type IV renal tubular acidosis)	Depolarising muscle paralysis
Pseudohypoaldosteronism	
Dietary potassium excess including prescribed supplements and upper gastrointestinal bleeding (with reduced renal clearance)	Hyperkalaemic periodic paralysis

Table 7.4 Causes of hyperkalaemia.

Management

Firstly, dietary potassium intake should be restricted; **Table 7.5** lists the main sources of dietary potassium.

Emergency management This is required at plasma potassium >6.3 mmol/L, due to risk of arrhythmia. If the ECG is abnormal, 10 mL of 10% calcium gluconate or calcium chloride is given slowly intravenously (at a maximum rate of 2 mL/min), repeating the dose if necessary 30–60 minutes later, to stabilise the myocardium and prevent arrhythmias.

Insulin Insulin can be used to drive potassium out of the plasma into cells, 10–20 units of soluble insulin with 50 mL 50%

	Significant >0.25 g (6.25 mmol)/100 g	**High** >0.5 g (12.5 mmol)/100 g	**Very high** >1 g (25 mmol)/100 g
Vegetables	Potato		Seaweed
	Carrot		
	Spinach		
	Broccoli		
	Butternut squash		
	Beetroot		
	Cauliflower		
	Mushroom		
Fruits	Banana	Dried fruit (raisins, dates, prunes)	Dried figs/apricots
	Orange		
	Melon	Nuts	
	Kiwi	Avocado	
	Blackcurrant		
	Plum		
	Tomato		
Pulses	Baked beans		Soya flour
	Kidney beans		
	Lentils		
Meat	Beef		
	Pork		
	Lamb		
	Poultry		
	Fish		
Grains		Bran cereals	
		Wheat germ	
Other		Chocolate	Molasses
			Coffee (instant)
			Lo-salt (12 mmol K^+/g as potassium chloride)

Table 7.5 Potassium-rich foods. Modified from Gennari FJ. Hypokalemia. *New Engl J Med* 1998; 339: 451–458.

glucose (or equivalent as 20% glucose which is less sclerosant to veins). If hyperkalaemia persists after a few hours, the infusion can be repeated. The blood glucose should be checked every hour.

Intravenous sodium bicarbonate In severely acidotic patients correction of the acidosis using intravenous sodium bicarbonate may allow the exchange of potassium ions for hydrogen ions across the cell membrane. β-adrenergic agonists will lower the plasma potassium concentration in many patients but 20–40% experience only a modest reduction (<0.5 mmol/L). The use of oral ion exchange resins for the treatment of hyperkalaemia is a standard clinical practice although the evidence in support of efficacy is rather weak. Uncontrollable hyperkalaemia in a patient with renal impairment is an indication for renal replacement therapy.

Clinical insight

Severe hyperkalaemia is a medical emergency requiring immediate management, as there is a significant risk of cardiac arrest.

Prognosis and complications

The most dangerous complication of hyperkalaemia is cardiac arrest with asystole or ventricular fibrillation.

7.6 Hypocalcaemia and hypercalcaemia

Overview of calcium homeostasis

Ionised calcium that is free in plasma is the physiologically relevant component and comprises approximately 50% of total plasma calcium. Total plasma calcium is usually maintained in the narrow range of 2.1–2.5 mmol/L. Synthesis of active vitamin D depends on the addition of a 1-hydroxy group to 25-hydroxy vitamin D in the kidney. Renal damage results in reduced synthesis of active 1,25 hydroxy vitamin D3 with a tendency to hypocalcaemia through reduced intestinal calcium absorption.

The resulting hypocalcaemia, as well as the phosphate retention due to a reduced GFR, stimulate the secretion of parathyroid hormone (PTH). This mobilises calcium from the bones contributing to renal osteodystrophy and over time can evolve from secondary to tertiary hyperparathyroidism where failure to respond to the normal regulatory feedback mechanism results in hypercalcaemia. The combination of hypercalcaemia and high plasma phosphate can lead to calcium deposition at a number of sites, including the skin and blood vessels.

Hypocalcaemia
Causes
Alkalosis, e.g. due to prolonged hyperventilation can lead to functional hypocalcaemia due to a fall in the ionized plasma Ca^{2+} concentration. Causes of a fall in total plasma Ca^{2+} include: primary hypoparathyroidism, renal failure, vitamin D deficiency and malabsorption, acute pancreatitis, rhabdomyolysis and sepsis. Low plasma Mg^{2+} can also cause hypocalcaemia without any change in total body calcium.

Clinical features
Hypocalcaemia causes increased neuromuscular activity with:
- Paraesthesia
- Muscle cramps
- Carpopedal spasm
- In extreme cases: tetany, laryngeal stridor and convulsions
- Positive Chvostek and Trousseau signs of tetany may be elicited

These effects are determined by the concentration of ionised calcium and are influenced by plasma pH (available calcium concentration falls the more alkaline the plasma).

Investigations
Serum creatinine and electrolytes, albumin, phosphate, 1,25-hydroxyvitamin D and magnesium, blood glucose and plasma PTH should be measured. A full blood count and ECG should be carried out.

Management
Attempts to raise the available calcium should be made if the plasma 'adjusted' calcium is <1.8 mmol/L or the patient has unequivocal signs of hypocalcaemia.

$$\text{Adjusted calcium (mmol/L)} = \text{unadjusted calcium (mmol/L)} +$$
$$0.02 \times (40 - \text{serum albumin (g/L)})$$

Calcium supplements These can be given by mouth along with vitamin D replacement.

> ### Clinical insight
>
> Intravenous calcium is sclerosant (i.e. causes inflammation and subsequent fibrosis) and great care should be taken to avoid extravasation from veins. Calcium solutions should be administered via as large a vein as possible.

Calcium gluconate If urgent replacement is indicated, 10 mL of 10% calcium gluconate (2.2 mmol Ca^{2+}), no faster than 2 mL/min should be given intravenously. The effect is short-lasting so the infusion should be followed by intravenous calcium gluconate 10%, 40 mL (in 500 mL 0.9% NaCl or 5% dextrose) over 24 hours. This will provide 8.8 mmol of Ca^{2+}.

Monitoring The Ca^{2+} concentration should be measured three to four times daily until serum Ca^{2+} is within the normal range, adjusting the infusion rate as appropriate.

Hypomagnesaemic hypocalcaemia This should be treated with intravenous magnesium alone.

Prognosis and complications
Clinical features usually resolve with restoration of normal plasma calcium concentration. Chronic hypocalcaemia may contribute to the development of osteomalacia.

Hypercalcaemia
Causes
Hypercalcaemia can occur as a result of reduced excretion, increased absorption or a shift of calcium between body compartments. Common causes are primary hyperparathyroidism, thiazide diuretics and malignant disease (particularly myeloma, lung or breast cancer, lymphoma). Rarer causes include sarcoidosis, thyrotoxicosis, vitamin D intoxication, calcium-containing drugs, cortisol deficiency and familial hypocalciuric hypercalcaemia.

Clinical features

Hypercalcaemia may produce no symptoms or can cause thirst, polyuria (due to nephrogenic diabetes insipidus), nausea, vomiting, constipation and abdominal pain. There may be confusion or coma.

Investigations

Ideally, calcium should be checked on an uncuffed blood sample, to avoid the haemoconcentration and falsely raised total calcium caused by venepuncture with a tourniquet. Serum creatinine and electrolytes, phosphate, albumin, alkaline phosphatase and plasma PTH should be measured. Other tests that should be done are: thyroid blood tests, full blood count, chest X-ray, ECG, serum and urine protein electrophoresis if myeloma suspected, erythrocyte sedimentation rate and C-reactive protein.

Management

An attempt should be made to lower the serum calcium in anyone with an 'adjusted' serum calcium of >3 mmol/L unless the value is stable and the patient completely asymptomatic (for calculation of adjusted calcium see section on hypocalcaemia).

Drugs that contain calcium or cause hypercalcaemia (e.g. thiazide diuretics) should be discontinued.

Fluids Patients with hypercalcaemia are usually volume deplete, and this should be corrected with 0.9% NaCl aiming to increase urine volume to 200 mL/h to promote calciuresis. Consider giving furosemide (40–80 mg orally or intravenously) to increase urine flow and calciuresis, ensuring that the patient is not rendered hypovolaemic. Regular clinical assessment of volume status is essential.

Bisphosphonate If the serum calcium is still high after 24 hours, intravenous bisphosphonate should be given. The serum calcium should fall within 24–48 hours with the maximum response taking 4–5 days.

Hyperparathyroidism Chronic hypercalcaemia due to primary or tertiary hyperparathyroidism may require parathyroidectomy, with use of the calcimimetic cinacalcet as an alternative for tertiary hyperparathyroidism.

Prognosis and complications

Prognosis depends on the aetiology. Persistent hypercalcaemia associated with hyperphosphataemia leads to vascular calcification, which is a factor in the high rate of cardiovascular morbidity and mortality in patients with chronic kidney disease.

Acid–base disorders

Buffering challenges

The body's acid–base balance as measured by the blood pH is tightly controlled. When either acidosis or alkalosis develops, many of the body's functions (both cellular and organs) will be impaired. The blood pH is usually within the range 7.35–7.45. Challenging the balance is the production of acid from both metabolism (carbonic acid) and by-products of our dietary intake (e.g. sulphuric acid, phosphoric acid). Buffering mechanisms to maintain the balance in the face of wide variations in the rate of acid production include:

- The bicarbonate/carbonic acid system
- Proteins in cells
- Haemoglobin
- Bones

In the short term, it is the bicarbonate system that is the most important. When this buffering system is unable to cope, acidosis or alkalosis develops. The terminology for acid–base disorders is difficult to understand, but understanding three key principles should help you:

- Henderson–Hasselbalch equation
- Compensation
- Acid–base states

The Henderson–Hasselbalch equation

The relationship between pH, hydrogen ions and carbon dioxide in the body is described by the Henderson–Hasselbalch equation. Carbonic anhydrase is the enzyme which catalyses the following reactions to try to ensure that a balance is maintained:

$$H^+ + HCO_3^- \Leftrightarrow H_2CO_3 \Leftrightarrow H_2O + CO_2$$

Compensation

The lungs and kidneys can manipulate the body's levels of carbon dioxide and bicarbonate, respectively, and in doing so can influence the buffering mechanism and hence the blood pH. This is called compensation and can either be respiratory (i.e. lung) or metabolic (i.e. kidney).

Acid–base states

The blood pH, bicarbonate and partial pressure of carbon dioxide (PCO_2) can be used to define four acid–base states:

- Metabolic acidosis
- Metabolic alkalosis
- Respiratory acidosis
- Respiratory alkalosis

8.1 Clinical scenarios

Intense metabolic acidosis

Presentation

An 89-year-old man is brought to the emergency department after being found collapsed at home. He has a reduced level of consciousness and is hyperventilating.

Immediate management

The initial assessment includes a rapid review of the airway, breathing and circulation, and Glasgow Coma Scale, as well as basic investigations such as a blood sugar. This assessment may identify clinical problems that need to be addressed urgently. High-flow oxygen is given to the patient via a facemask and non-rebreathe bag.

Further history

The ambulance crew inform the emergency team that the patient may have been on the floor of his kitchen for two days.

Examination

His respiratory rate is 36 breaths/min and he appears volume deplete, with a low jugular venous pressure (JVP), blood pressure 82/46 mm Hg and cool peripheries.

Investigations

His capillary blood sugar is normal. Urea and electrolytes show a raised creatinine concentration of 870 µmol/L (normal range

60–110), sodium 136 mmol/L and potassium 6.8 mmol/L. His creatine kinase is found to be 140,000 U/L. An arterial blood gas taken while he is on 10 L oxygen per minute shows a pH 7.1, PO_2 24 kPa, PCO_2 2.4 kPa, bicarbonate 13 mmol/L. His electrocardiogram (ECG) demonstrates wide QRS complexes and peaked T waves. A urine sample is noted to be smoky brown in appearance and urinalysis identifies blood in the urine.

Diagnostic approach

The low pH and low bicarbonate suggest that he has a metabolic acidosis. His PCO_2 is low due to respiratory compensation as the body tries to excrete CO_2 to maintain the acid–base balance through the bicarbonate buffering system. The raised creatinine and potassium suggests that the cause may be an acute kidney injury. The most probable cause is rhabdomyolysis as the creatine kinase is elevated and the blood in the urine is likely to be a false positive from myoglobin.

Treatment

The life-threatening hyperkalaemia is initially treated medically with 10 mL of 10% calcium gluconate and a dextrose insulin infusion. The patient is transferred to the intensive care unit for monitoring. Despite fluid resuscitation he needs renal replacement therapy to control the acid–base balance and hyperkalaemia.

Nausea and vomiting for 48 hours

Presentation

A 46-year-old man with nausea and vomiting for the past 48 hours is referred to the medical team by his general practitioner.

Examination

He is hypotensive with a blood pressure of 98/55 mm Hg and a respiratory rate of 9 breaths/min.

Investigations

Blood tests sent by the emergency team include blood gases (pH 7.48, PO_2 9.8 kPa, PCO_2 6.8 kPa, bicarbonate 33 mmol/L). The potassium is 2.3 mmol/L (low).

Diagnostic approach

Vomiting causes a loss of acid (hydrochloric acid) from the stomach. If this is prolonged the blood gas analysis can show alkalosis. The high bicarbonate suggests that this patient has metabolic alkalosis. The PCO_2 may rise through respiratory compensation but hypoxia will limit this by preventing hypoventilation.

Investigation

Gastric losses result in the loss of hydrochloric acid and therefore a low serum chloride can confirm the diagnosis of a metabolic alkalosis secondary to gastric losses.

8.2 Metabolic acidosis

Clinical features

In the acute setting the patient is often unwell and hyper-ventilating. Hyperventilation is an attempt to blow off acid via carbon dioxide excretion. The resulting hyperventilation is called Kussmaul's breathing.

Investigation

Metabolic acidosis (pH <7.35) occurs in one of three settings:
- Generation of an excess of hydrogen ions that cannot be excreted fast enough (e.g. acute kidney injury, diabetic ketoacidosis, lactic acidosis)
- Loss of bicarbonate (e.g. diarrhoea)
- Ingestion of acidic substances (e.g. ethanol, salicylates, ethylene glycol)

Arterial blood gas will show:
- ↓ Blood pH
- ↓ Bicarbonate
- ↓ PCO_2 (respiratory compensation)

Calculating the anion gap (**Table 8.1**) can be useful in evaluating the cause. To do this, the serum chloride needs to be determined. Usually this must be requested specifically from biochemistry or may be shown by some blood gas machines.

Normal anion gap	Increased anion gap
Bicarbonate loss (e.g. diarrhoea, ileostomy, ureterosigmoidostomy, proximal renal tubular acidosis, hypoaldosteronism)	Renal failure
Reduced renal H^+ excretion (e.g. distal renal tubular acidosis)	Lactic acidosis
	Ketoacidosis (e.g. diabetic ketoacidosis, starvation, enzyme deficiencies)
	Intoxication (e.g. methanol, ethylene glycol, ethanol, salicylates, paraldehyde)

Table 8.1 Causes of normal or increased anion gap metabolic acidosis.

$$\text{Anion gap} = [Na^+ + K^+] - [Cl^- + HCO_3^-]$$

In health, the anion gap is usually between 8 and 17 mmol/L. If there is hypoalbuminaemia, caution is needed in interpreting the anion gap, as hypoalbuminaemia itself lowers the anion gap. Having calculated the anion gap other specific tests such as a blood sugar, lactate or drug levels may be appropriate.

Management

Treatment depends on identifying the underlying cause. After senior review in a high dependency environment the use of intravenous sodium bicarbonate can be useful in the following types of metabolic acidosis:

- Life-threatening acidosis (pH <7.0, bicarbonate <10 mmol/L) to rebalance the bicarbonate/carbonic acid buffering system
- Renal failure and the treatment of severe hyperkalaemia
- Intoxication with salicylates, as it promotes excretion

Additional carbon dioxide is generated when sodium bicarbonate is given, and ventilatory reserves must be adequate, otherwise the patient's clinical state will worsen due to respiratory failure.

A chronic mild metabolic acidosis may be treated with oral sodium bicarbonate.

8.3 Metabolic alkalosis

Clinical features

These can vary. The elevated pH reduces the free serum calcium and this can lead to tingling, paraesthesia, tetany and convulsions. The majority of causes are associated with volume depletion, e.g. low jugular venous pressure, low blood pressure and reduced urine output.

Investigation

Arterial blood gas will show:
- ↑ Blood pH
- ↑ Bicarbonate
- (Often normal) PCO_2

The kidney can normally rapidly excrete excess bicarbonate, therefore one of two factors is usually present that is stopping this bicarbonate loss (**Table 8.2**):
- Chloride deficiency: as chloride and bicarbonate are the major anions in the extracellular fluid, when there is chloride deficiency the kidney reabsorbs more bicarbonate to maintain the electroneutrality of the extracellular fluid

Low chloride	Low potassium	Other
Gastrointestinal losses (e.g. vomiting, villous adenoma)	Renal tubular disorders	Milk alkali syndrome
Drugs (e.g. diuretics)	Drugs (e.g. laxatives)	Drugs (e.g. bicarbonate supplementation, penicillins)
Cystic fibrosis	Hyperaldosteronism (e.g. primary, secondary from liquorice ingestion)	

Table 8.2 Causes of metabolic alkalosis.

- Potassium depletion: bicarbonate reabsorption in the kidney increases in the presence of potassium depletion

Usually the cause is apparent from the history and examination. In those who are not on diuretics a spot urinary chloride will help distinguish those who are volume deplete (low urinary chloride) compared with those who are euvolaemic or who have volume expansion (normal or high urinary chloride). ECG changes similar to those seen in hypokalaemia can be present (i.e. prominent U waves).

Chloride depletion is the most common association in clinical practice (>90% cases). It occurs in vomiting and loss of gastric secretions via nasogastric tubes (through loss of hydrochloric acid) and diuretic use (interference with the reabsorption of sodium and chloride in renal tubules).

There can be some respiratory compensation for metabolic alkalosis but this is limited by the drive to prevent hypoxia. Hypoventilation and elevation of the PCO_2 beyond 7 kPa is rarely seen.

Management

In the majority of causes (chloride deficiency and volume depletion) the treatment will be intravenous fluids containing chloride (i.e. 0.9% sodium chloride). Where potassium depletion is present, the patient will need potassium supplementation. In all cases where an underlying precipitant is identified, if possible, this should be addressed (i.e. gastric outflow obstruction treated, villous adenoma removed, diuretics stopped).

8.4 Respiratory acidosis

Clinical features

Respiratory acidosis occurs when there is hypoventilation leading to an increase in PCO_2. Hypercapnia (high PCO_2) will increase intracerebral pressure, increase peripheral and cerebral blood flow (by vasodilatation) and stimulate ventilation, leading to the clinical features:

- Dyspnoea

- Confusion/reduced consciousness
- Headache
- Warm and flushed
- Tachycardic with a characteristic bounding pulse

Investigation

A chest X-ray may be diagnostic for some of the common causes such as pneumonia, pneumothorax, pulmonary oedema, lung diseases including asthma, and inadequate mechanical ventilation in those on ventilator support.

Other less common mechanisms of hypoventilation include:

- Central nervous system disorders (e.g. stroke, respiratory depression by drugs)
- Neuromuscular problems (e.g. myasthenia gravis)
- Chest wall deformities (e.g. trauma)
- Catabolic (e.g. malignant hyperthermia)
- Iatrogenic causes (absorption of carbon dioxide following carbon dioxide insufflation into a body cavity for laparoscopic surgery)

Arterial blood gas will show:

- $\downarrow$ Blood pH
- $\uparrow$ Bicarbonate (metabolic compensation)
- $\uparrow PCO_2$

Over the course of days, the kidney can increase H^+ excretion and as a result the Henderson–Hasselbalch equation shifts to the left and serum bicarbonate concentration becomes elevated.

Management

Treatment of the underlying pathology is needed. Some patients may require respiratory support in the form of either non-invasive ventilation or intubation.

8.5 Respiratory alkalosis

Clinical features

Hyperventilation must occur for respiratory alkalosis to develop; the patient will have a high respiratory rate. A common presentation of psychogenic hyperventilation is paraesthesia of extremities and lips (alkalosis induced fall of ionised calcium) and chest discomfort.

Investigation

Hyperventilation arises either in response to hypoxia (e.g. asthma, pneumonia or pulmonary oedema) or states that increase central respiratory drive (e.g. pregnancy, anxiety). It is therefore important to exclude or treat hypoxia early.
Arterial blood gas will show:

- ↑ Blood pH
- ↓ Bicarbonate (metabolic compensation)
- ↓ PCO_2

The increased alveolar ventilation will lower the PCO_2, which is detected by central and peripheral chemoreceptors and will limit hyperventilation in most cases. Two mechanisms result in a fall in bicarbonate:

- HCO_3^- converts to CO_2 which is excreted by the lung
- Increased excretion of bicarbonate by the kidney (metabolic compensation)

Management

Treatment is directed towards the underlying precipitant. Other than the effects of the alkalosis on the ionised calcium, the clinical consequence of respiratory alkalosis is reduced cerebral blood flow and therefore a fall in intracerebral pressure. This can be used clinically in acute head injuries where hyperventilation induced by a ventilator can lower intracranial pressure.

8.6 Mixed pictures

The clinical history and examination should allow you to anticipate the most likely acid–base status in the majority of cases, and the blood gas analysis and biochemistry will confirm or refute your hypothesis. Sometimes, the acid–base status suggests that a further problem exists, e.g. you may anticipate that a patient with new-onset diabetes who has a high respiratory rate is likely to have an increased anion gap metabolic acidosis (low pH, low PCO_2 and low HCO_3) as a result of diabetic ketoacidosis. However, if they also have pneumonia then the respiratory compensation will be inadequate and so they may also have a respiratory acidosis. Depending on the severity, the change in PCO_2 and HCO_3^- may be partially overturned or reversed.

A series of rules and nomograms exist and may be helpful in these more complex situations.

Hypertension

Hypertension is a clinical condition of elevated pressure in the arteries, due to:

- Abnormalities of the vessel wall which increase peripheral vascular resistance

and/or

- Fluid retention which increases cardiac output

The increased pressure causes injury both to the blood vessel itself, and also to the organs supplied, such as the heart, brain, eyes and kidneys. Hypertension affects a large portion of the adult population. It is often undiagnosed and hence untreated; as a result it is a major contributor to excess morbidity and mortality on a worldwide basis.

9.1 Clinical scenarios

First diagnosis of hypertension in middle age

Presentation

A 50-year-old Caucasian man on a routine check-up with his general practitioner is found to have a blood pressure of 165/90 mmHg.

Diagnostic approach

Blood pressure is recorded as the mean of 3 measurements, to reduce the impact of patient anxiety and operator bias.

Further history/examination

On further questioning, he has no symptoms and has been recorded as having a normal blood pressure during a gallbladder operation when he was 30 years of age. He is a non-smoker and consumes 10 units of alcohol weekly. His body mass index (BMI) is 31 kg/m²; the rest of his physical examination, including funduscopy, is normal.

Diagnostic approach

In order to assess any damage to target organs, urine examination, electrocardiography (ECG) and renal function blood tests are performed.

Investigations

The urine dipstick examination shows trace proteinuria, and the ECG demonstrates left ventricular hypertrophy. Blood tests show a reduced estimated glomerular filtration rate (eGFR).

Diagnostic approach

This patient has evidence of injury to both his kidneys and heart, indicating longstanding hypertension. His management plan includes advice to do regular exercise, lose weight, and reduce salt in his diet, and he is started on ramipril, an angiotensin-converting enzyme (ACE) inhibitor.

Diabetes and high blood pressure

Presentation

A 75-year-old man is referred to the diabetic clinic with a rising serum creatinine concentration and proteinuria. His eGFR has decreased by 4 mL/min/1.73 m^2 over the previous six months. He has no angina or leg cramps, and has never had a cerebrovascular accident. He is found to have background diabetic retinopathy. His blood pressure is 138/85 mmHg and he is taking 10 mg amlodipine once a day. His urine albumin/creatinine ratio is 54 mg/mmol (normal <3).

Diagnostic approach

Given the evidence of diabetic microvascular disease in the retina, this patient almost certainly has diabetic nephropathy. Renal biopsy is not usually necessary in this situation, and would only be considered if there were unusual features, such as the absence of microvascular disease elsewhere, haematuria or a rapid deterioration in eGFR.

Further management

The key aspect in managing diabetic nephropathy is excellent control of blood pressure, targeting <130/80 mmHg, using

ACEis or angiotensin II receptor blockers. Lisinopril was therefore added to his medication. Three months later hydrochlorothiazide was added as a combination pill with lisinopril to achieve a blood pressure <130/80 mmHg. The rate of decrease in eGFR slowed, and was 2 mL/min/1.73 m² over the next six months; proteinuria also decreased.

9.2 Primary hypertension

The term primary hypertension describes raised blood pressure for which there is no apparent cause; it is also known as idiopathic or essential hypertension.

Hypertension in the general population is defined as a persistent elevation of blood pressure >140 mmHg systolic and 90 mmHg diastolic. One single high reading can be misleading: therefore, at any examination blood pressure should be measured at least twice, or until 2 readings are obtained with systolic pressures within 5 mmHg. Ranges of blood pressure are:

- Normal blood pressure: <120/80 mmHg
- Pre-hypertension is >120/80 mmHg and <139/89 mmHg
- Severe hypertension: >160/100 mmHg

Individuals with pre-hypertension are prone to develop hypertension and hence need follow-up. Severe hypertension requires immediate management. **Table 9.1** shows the definition and classification of elevated blood pressure.

	Office blood pressure (BP) (mmHg)		Ambulatory BP (mmHg)
	Systolic BP	Diastolic BP	
Normal BP	<120	<80	
Pre-hypertension	120–139	80–90	
Stage 1	140–159	90–99	≥135/85
Stage 2	≥160	≥100	
Isolated systolic	≥140	<90	

Table 9.1 Definition and stages of hypertension.

Epidemiology

Hypertension is the commonest reversible risk factor for cardio-vascular morbidity and mortality. High blood pressure affects about a third of the adult population in North America and Europe: in the USA 29.9% of adults are affected, and in the UK in 2010 the prevalence of hypertension was 30%, of which only 10% were well controlled. The prevalence increases with age.

Pathogenesis

There are several mechanisms by which pressure increases in blood vessels. Pressure is determined by the force and volume of blood pumped out by the heart, and the resistance to the flow in the arterial vessels. Hence, blood pressure is the product of cardiac output and peripheral resistance (i.e. blood pressure = cardiac output × peripheral resistance).

The proposed causes of essential or primary hypertension involve mechanisms by which either cardiac output and/or peripheral resistance is increased, as discussed below (**Figure 9.1**).

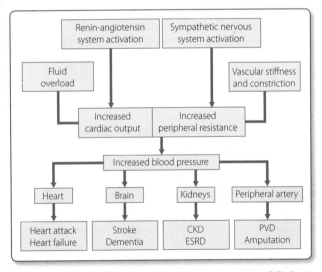

Figure 9.1 The mechanism of hypertension and target organ injury. CKD, chronic kidney disease . ESRD, end-stage renal disease. PVD, peripheral vascular disease.

Renin–angiotensin system Activation of the renin–angiotensin system (**Figure 9.2**; see also **Figure 1.7**) increases blood pressure by an increase in both peripheral resistance and blood volume. Renin is an aspartyl protease secreted from the juxtaglomerular apparatus (JGA) in the kidney in response to low sodium chloride delivery to the tubular lumen, low systemic blood pressure or sympathetic stimulation.

1. Renin cleaves angiotensin to angiotensin I, which is a decapeptide
2. Angiotensin I is further cleaved by ACE, predominantly in the lungs, to angiotensin II, an octapeptide
3. Angiotensin II causes vasoconstriction by binding to angiotensin II type I receptors in the blood vessel wall, thereby increasing peripheral resistance
4. Angiotensin II also causes release of aldosterone from the adrenal medulla, which in turn acts on the renal tubules to enhance salt and water retention, thereby increasing blood volume

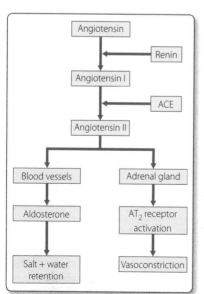

Figure 9.2 The renin–angiotensin system and hypertension. ACE, angiotensin-converting enzyme.

Other effects of the system include:

- Inactivation of the vasodilator protein bradykinin by ACE
- Over a period of time, stimulation of vascular smooth muscle cell growth by angiotensin II, causing vascular remodelling with a permanent increase in peripheral resistance.

Sympathetic nervous system Activation of the sympathetic nervous system increases blood pressure principally by increasing peripheral resistance through activation of the α_1 receptors on vascular small muscle cells, mainly by the hormone norepinephrine and to a lesser extent epinephrine. Stimulation of the β_1 receptors in the heart increases cardiac contractility and heart rate, thereby increasing cardiac output. β_1 receptor stimulation in the kidney also causes renin release, thereby activating the renin–angiotensin system as discussed above.

> ### Clinical insight
>
> Negative feedback control of norepinephrine release at the synaptic junction in the sympathetic system is maintained by the action of norepinephrine on α_2 receptors on the presynaptic junction. α_2 adrenergic agonist antihypertensive drugs (e.g. clonidine) lower blood pressure by stimulating these presynaptic α_2 receptors.

Intravascular volume An increase in the intravascular volume due to salt and water retention contributes to elevation of blood pressure; excess salt intake with food, or a decreased ability of the kidney to excrete excess salt, can cause this increase in blood volume. Intrinsic kidney disease, and activation of other hormonal pathways as described above, decreases the ability of the kidney to excrete salt.

Blood vessel changes Structural and functional abnormalities of blood vessels can cause increased blood pressure. In young hypertensive patients, hypertrophy of medium-sized arteries increases peripheral resistance. In elderly patients increased stiffness of central arteries increases systolic blood pressure, causing isolated systolic hypertension.

Vascular smooth muscle and endothelial cells are major determinants of blood pressure: endothelial cells release mediators which cause constriction and relaxation of vascular smooth muscle cells, regulating blood flow to the periphery. Dysfunctional endothelial cells disproportionately release vasoconstrictors and thereby increase blood pressure. Vasoconstriction is also caused by abnormal ion transport mechanisms in the cells of the vascular wall.

Clinical features

High blood pressure is often diagnosed at a routine check-up. Most patients are asymptomatic when diagnosed, although occasionally patients complain of headaches. However, patients may present with features of complications as detailed below.

Complications

Heart Hypertension is a major risk factor for ischaemic heart disease: it is associated with increased atherosclerosis and hence acute coronary syndromes. The heart in hypertension has to pump against an increased resistance, which causes thickening of the left ventricular wall, left ventricular stiffening and, with time, left ventricular diastolic and systolic dysfunction. The left atrium dilates due the pressure transmitted from the left ventricular cavity. The dilated left atrium is prone to arrhythmias. Hence, hypertension is associated with atrial fibrillation and congestive heart failure.

Kidney Hypertension causes kidney disease over time. Elevated blood pressure is a major determinant of progression of chronic kidney disease due to other causes, such as diabetes, often resulting in end-stage kidney failure. The early clinical feature of hypertensive kidney disease is proteinuria; it takes considerable time for elevated systolic blood pressure to cause a decrease in GFR.

As mentioned, hypertension is a risk factor for atherosclerosis, which can also contribute to renal dysfunction by causing stenosis of both large and small renal arteries.

Brain Stroke due to elevated blood pressure remains a major cause of mortality and morbidity in the general population. The risk increases with rising blood pressure, particularly systolic pressure, even when the levels are within the normal range. Hypertension is also associated with an increased risk of dementia. Occasionally, very high blood pressure can cause hypertensive encephalopathy, manifested as confusion, focal signs, seizures and, ultimately, coma.

Peripheral arteries High blood pressure is associated with peripheral vascular disease, manifesting most commonly as lower limb ischaemia.

Investigations

Correct assessment of blood pressure is essential for diagnosis and the management of hypertension. Blood pressure can be measured at the clinic, at home or continuously monitored during the day. Blood pressure should ideally be measured:

- With a regularly calibrated machine
- With a cuff of appropriate size
- After 15 minutes of rest
- In a sitting position
- With the arm supported at the level of the heart
- After avoidance of tea, coffee or smoking for at least 30 minutes prior to measurement

Causes of secondary hypertension may also need to be investigated if indicated (see Section 9.3).

Clinical insight

Multiple home blood pressure readings and 24-hour ambulatory blood pressure readings are more reliable and often necessary to make an accurate diagnosis. They are sometimes also used to monitor patients and guide further management.

Management

Treatment of hypertension is associated with a major reduction in the incidence of myocardial infarction, stroke and end-stage renal disease, diseases which consume a major share of healthcare resources. Every effort, therefore, should be made to diagnose and treat hypertension.

Hypertension is often asymptomatic, and hence diagnosed late. Due to the lack of symptoms, it is sometimes difficult to convince patients to embark on lifelong therapy. Lifestyle modifications (**Table 9.2**) should be tried in all patients, and this is dependent on good patient education and motivation.

Dietary salt restriction	<6 gm salt day
Weight restriction	Aim for body mass index <25 kg/m²
Increase physical activity	>30 min day
Decrease alcohol intake	<2unit/day (men) and <1 unit/day (women)
Improve diet	Increase fruit and vegetable intake; less saturated fat

Table 9.2 Lifestyle change advice for management of hypertension.

Medication Where blood pressure is initially very high, or is high and either associated with target organ damage or not controlled by lifestyle modifications, medication should be commenced. The choice of antihypertensive is guided by a patient's age and ethnicity, and is added in steps until satisfactory control is achieved. The National Institute for Health and Clinical Excellence and the British Hypertension Society in the UK advise the following steps (**Figure 9.3**):

> **Clinical insight**
>
> The key to effective management of hypertension is a good patient–doctor relationship. Patient education in order to understand the consequences of elevated blood pressure is key to their motivation for managing it.

1. Patients under the age of 55 years with stage 2 or above hypertension should be started on an ACE inhibitor; those above the age of 55 years of age, or a person of African or Caribbean origin of any age, should be started on a calcium channel blocker
2. If the target blood pressure is not reached, an ACE inhibitor or calcium channel blocker is added
3. A thiazide-like diuretic is added
4. 'Resistant hypertension' – an α-blocker or β-blocker is considered (see **Table 9.3** for a list of commonly used drugs and their doses).

> **Clinical insight**
>
> Patients should be advised that antihypertensive medication is usually lifelong, and can be associated with side effects, such as weakness, tiredness, dizziness, nausea, ankle swelling (with calcium channel blockers) and cough (ACE inhibitors).

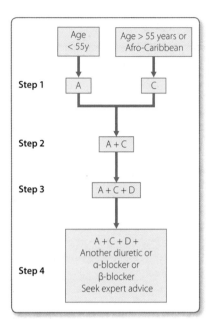

Figure 9.3 Stepwise management of hypertension. A, angiotensin-converting enzyme inhibitor or angiotensin receptor blocker. C, calcium channel blocker. D, diuretic.

Hypertension in diabetes Hypertension is a major cause of macro-and microvascular disease in patients with long-standing diabetes. Control of blood pressure to lower levels (<130/80 mmHg) is necessary to slow the progression of nephropathy, retinopathy, neuropathy and, to some extent, coronary artery and cerebrovascular disease. Inhibition of the renin–angiotensin system provides additional advantages; hence the use of ACE inhibitors and angiotensin receptor blockers is associated with better outcomes than other antihypertensive agents. For example, in the second clinical scenario above, the rate of declining eGFR was reduced from 4 to 2 mL/min/m^2 over six months with good control of blood pressure and use of an ACE inhibitor.

Prognosis

Uncontrolled hypertension leads to the complications detailed above. However, the course of the disease with respect to target organ injury can be significantly changed with proper

Drug	Dose
Angiotensin-converting enzyme (ACE) inhibitor	
Ramipril	2.5–10 mg OD
Lisinopril	5–20 mg OD
Calcium channel blocker	
Amlodipine	5–10 mg OD
Nifedipine, long acting	30–90 mg OD
β-blocker	
Atenolol	25–50 mg OD
Metoprolol	25–100 mg BD
Angiotensin II receptor blocker	
Losartan	25–100 mg OD
Irbesartan	75–300 mg OD
Diuretic	
Bendroflumethiazide	2.5 mg OD
Chlorthalidone	25–50 mg OD
Others	
Doxazosin	2–8 mg BD
Hydralazine	25–50 mg BD

Table 9.3 Commonly used antihypertensive agents. BD, twice daily. OD, once daily.

management. Lowering blood pressure, even if not to ideal goals, reduces the incidence of stroke and myocardial ischaemia, and prolongs survival.

9.3 Secondary hypertension

Hypertension is sometimes a result of renal, renovascular or endocrine causes. These conditions are far less common than primary hypertension, occurring in less than 5% of patients with hypertension.

If suspected, the secondary cause should be diagnosed, as it can alter management, and in some cases lead to a cure. For example, renal artery stenosis due to fibromuscular dysplasia in a young person can be treated with renal artery dilatation and stenting. A Conn adenoma, causing elevated blood pressure due to increased secretion of aldosterone, can be cured with laparoscopic removal of the tumour. The common causes of secondary hypertension and relevant diagnostic methods are listed in **Table 9.4**.

Renovascular hypertension

Hypertension due to stenosis of one or both of the renal arteries is seen in young adults with fibromuscular dysplasia, and in patients above the age of 55 years with atherosclerotic disease, commonly at the ostium of the artery. The index of suspicion for renovascular hypertension is high in younger (<30 years) or older (>55 years) patients, and when blood pressure is difficult to control.

Causes of secondary hypertension	Investigations (finding)
Renal parenchymal disease	Urine (protein, blood), blood (creatinine), ultrasound scan (bilateral small kidneys)
Renovascular disease	Ultrasound scan (asymmetrical kidneys), renal artery angiogram (stenosis)
Conn syndrome	Blood (high sodium, low potassium, high aldosterone, low renin), CT scan (adrenal adenoma)
Cushing syndrome	Blood (high sodium, low potassium, high cortisol), urine (high 24 h cortisol), CT scan (possible adrenal adenoma)
Phaeochromocytoma	Blood (high epinephrine, norepinephrinee) urine (increased 24 h catecholamines), CT scan (possible adrenal adenoma)

Table 9.4 Common causes of secondary hypertension and methods of diagnosis. CT, computed tomography.

Investigations

A renal artery angiogram using computed tomography (CT) or magnetic resonance imaging (MRI) is used to confirm the diagnosis.

Management

- In young patients with difficult-to-control hypertension, the best treatment is renal artery angioplasty, plus stenting if necessary
- In older patients, the results of angioplasty are not always beneficial and may indeed precipitate a sudden decline in renal function
- In selected older patients with deteriorating kidney function and difficult to control blood pressure, renal artery angioplasty may be beneficial in preventing progression of kidney disease and improving blood pressure control, but this is controversial

Hypertension in pregnancy

Elevated blood pressure during pregnancy can be due to chronic hypertension (essential and secondary), gestational hypertension and pre-eclampsia. Whatever the cause, hypertension can increase maternal and fetal complications and hence requires proper diagnosis, close monitoring, good blood pressure control and planning of delivery at the appropriate time.

Clinical features

By definition, chronic hypertension is present before pregnancy. However, the hypertension may not have been diagnosed, and can be masked due to the physiological dip in blood pressure that occurs in early pregnancy. Gestational hypertension usually presents with elevated blood pressure after 20 weeks of gestation without proteinuria. Both chronic hypertension and gestational hypertension carry the risk of developing pre-eclampsia, and treatment is initiated to keep the blood pressure <150/100 mmHg. Pre-eclampsia is associated with hypertension and proteinuria after 20 weeks of gestation.

Management
The goal of treatment is the safe delivery of a healthy baby, with blood pressure treated acutely only if >150–160 mmHg systolic and 100–100 mmHg diastolic. **Table 9.5** shows a list of safe antihypertensive drugs commonly used in pregnancy.

Hyperaldosteronism
Elevated aldosterone levels as a cause of resistant hypertension is not uncommon. Hypokalaemia and hypernatraemia are clues to the diagnosis but are not often found.

Diagnosis
Measurement of the renin/aldosterone ratio establishes the diagnosis: aldosterone concentration is high and renin concentration suppressed.

Management
Once the biochemical diagnosis is made, the adrenal glands should be imaged using CT or MRI. If a solitary adenoma is identified, removal of the adenoma using laparoscopic or open surgery can potentially cure hypertension. Bilateral adrenal hyperplasia is managed with agents such as spironolactone.

Oral	
α-methyldopa	250–500 TDS
Labetalol	100–400 BD
Nifedipine, long acting	30–60 mg OD
Intravenous	
Labetalol	50 mg over 1 min repeated after 5 min, max 200 mg
Hydralazine	50–200 μg/min

Table 9.5 Antihypertensives used in pregnancy. BD, twice daily. OD, once daily. TDS, three times daily.

9.4 Accelerated hypertension

Sudden elevations of blood pressure can be associated with acute target organ dysfunction such as:

- Heart failure
- Papilloedema
- Encephalopathy
- Stroke
- Renal failure

Due to routine examinations in primary care and the increased awareness of hypertension in the general population, cases of accelerated hypertension are now uncommon.

Management

These patients often require hospital admission and management of blood pressure with intravenous medications. It is important to remember not to lower blood pressure too quickly as this can jeopardise perfusion of organs such as the brain and kidney, which may have lost the capacity to autoregulate their blood flow. Intravenous medications commonly used include nitroglycerin, labetalol, hydralazine, nicardipine and sodium nitroprusside.

Tubulointerstitial disease

Structure and processing failure

The morphology of the glomerulus enables it to function as a structural filter. The filtrate from the glomerulus is selected mainly by molecular size. The tubules and interstitium, which make up 80% of the renal volume and are responsible for its architecture, then process the filtered load and have some endocrine roles seemingly out of keeping with their excretory function. The tubules selectively reabsorb or reject the filtrate to maintain the homeostasis of the internal milieu. The interstitium not only provides the scaffold for the tubules and glomeruli but also senses the degree of hypoxia in the cortex and produces erythropoietin as appropriate.

Disease of the tubules, therefore, whether primary (e.g. in a hereditary disorder such as Fanconi syndrome) or secondary to a systemic illness or toxicity, will cause a change in the concentration of a solute (plasma and/or urinary) or urine volume. Interstitial disease may produce anaemia or secondary effects from distortion of the renal architecture.

Tubulointerstitial disease

Tubulointerstitial disease, like glomerular disease, produces a limited set of responses to a wide range of initiating factors (**Table 10.1**). The changes seen are variable degrees of an inflammatory cell infiltrate, oedema, tubular separation and atrophy. A number of features point to interstitial disease:

- A clear history of a known drug toxin, e.g. ciclosporin, lithium, mesalazine, Chinese herbal remedies, compound analgesics
- Exposure to an infectious agent such as leptospirosis or hantavirus

Asymptomatic raised creatinine	Modest proteinuria (0.5 to 2 g/day or equivalent) Albumin level usually normal Oedema if fluid overloaded
Asymptomatic urinary abnormalities	Polyuria, glycosuria
Acute renal failure	Precipitating drug and decreased glomerular filtration rate developing over a few days
Progressive renal failure	As for acute renal, but over weeks and months
Chronic kidney disease	Typically small kidneys with modest haematuria/proteinuria

Table 10.1 Presentations of tubulointerstitial disease.

- Industrial exposure to metals such as lead
- Metabolic disorders such as hypercalcaemia or Wilson disease
- Systemic disorders such as Sjögren syndrome, sickle cell disease or light chain toxicities
- Regional localised disorders such as Balkan nephropathy
- Secondary to disorders such as reflux or obstructive uropathy
- Linked to other conditions such as uveitis but aetiology unknown, e.g. tubulointerstitial nephritis with uveitis (TINU) syndrome or sarcoidosis

Therefore, as with most renal conditions, a good history and detailed ultrasound imaging of the kidneys advances the differential diagnosis to a large extent.

10.1 Clinical scenario

Swollen legs

Presentation

A 75-year-old Caucasian man presents with moderate swelling of his legs. He first noted vague upper abdominal pains two weeks ago, and his appetite is reduced. Routine blood tests are sent.

Diagnostic approach

Peripheral oedema is a common and often a relative and non-specific finding, particularly in the elderly and in patients on calcium channel blockers. Recent onset and significant progression should prompt consideration of more serious underlying disease of the heart, liver or kidneys.

Further history

There is a significant past medical history of six years of Crohn colitis. The patient is on mesalazine, which he has been taking regularly for four years.

Examination

There is pitting oedema up to the mid-calf. No abnormalities are found on examination of the cardiovascular, respiratory or abdominal systems except for vague right upper quadrant tenderness.

Diagnostic approach

The lack of other significant history or findings on examination should prompt consideration of a diagnosis of a renal abnormality in this case. The urine should be tested; if there is proteinuria further renal investigations should be initiated.

Investigations

There is 2+ protein in the urine. Quantification gives a protein/creatinine ratio of 68 mg/mmol (normal <45). The patient's creatinine was normal when checked at the gastroenterological clinic nine months ago but is now 350 µmol/L.

Diagnostic approach

If any of the secondary causes of tubulointerstitial nephritis are suspected, the relevant investigations should be undertaken. If tubulointerstitial disease is suspected, renal

Clinical insight

Renal biopsy requires that the patient has two good-sized kidneys, normal clotting function, controlled blood pressure and is able to consent and cooperate with the procedure.

> ## Clinical insight
>
> A weakly positive antinuclear antibody (ANA), low level of paraproteinaemia or moderately raised rheumatoid factor are common in the elderly and should not stop the search for a more definitive diagnosis.

biopsy is required to make a histopathological diagnosis.

In this age group the differential diagnosis is wide and serological tests should be sent to look for a glomerular cause, and the urine analysed for casts and Bence Jones proteinuria. A biopsy is required to distinguish between these possibilities.

In this case, a renal biopsy shows interstitial nephritis.

10.2 Tubulointerstitial nephritis

The commonest aetiology of tubulointerstitial nephritis is drug related, but it can also be caused by certain infections and sarcoidosis. Many drugs are metabolised or excreted through the kidneys and it is this role that leads it to be susceptible to injury by these drugs.

Epidemiology

The geographical variation in the prevalence of this condition is based on the aetiological factors. Obvious examples include those living in the vicinity of a heavy metal smelting factory; a somewhat less obvious example is the link between high incidence of end-stage renal disease in Taiwan due to the popularity of Chinese herbal remedies.

Causes and pathogenesis

Tubulointerstitial nephritis is seen more commonly with some drugs than others (**Table 10.2**). However there are case reports of many other drugs being associated with this condition.

Two infections notable for inducing interstitial nephritis are hantavirus and leptospirosis, both associated with vectors which live near river water.

In most cases, the pathogenesis is not well understood. The exception to this is the immune-mediated mechanism in Sjögren syndrome and antitubular basement membrane disease.

5-aminosalicylates	For example, mesalazine (can occur anytime while on the drug not just after starting it)
Antibiotics	Classically meticillin, which is why it is no longer used clinically
	Ciprofloxacin
	Penicillins and cephalosporins
	Rifampicin
	Sulfonamides
Antiviral	Indinavir
Allopurinol	
Lithium	
Proton pump inhibitors	For example, omeprazole and lansoprazole

Table 10.2 The most frequently implicated drug causes of tubulointerstitial disease. There are reports of this condition with most drugs, however, some are widely prescribed (e.g. proton pump inhibitors), so that even a low frequency of tubulointerstitial disease occurring per prescription means they are seen more often than with prototypical drugs.

Clinical features

The condition should be considered when the history suggests a predisposing agent or conditions. Other suggestive features in the history are polyuria, nocturia (particularly prevalent in lithium-induced injury) and tubular dysfunction such as acidosis, glycosuria and amino aciduria.

Investigations

Urine The urine often contains both white and red cells with a low level of proteinuria (protein/creatinine ratio (PCR) <70). White cell casts are not often seen or looked for but have high specificity for the diagnosis of interstitial nephritis, as the interstitial inflammatory cells embed themselves in the Tamm–Horsfield protein secreted by the tubules.

Renal biopsy The gold standard test is renal biopsy, which enables identification of tubulointerstitial nephritis and the exclusion of a glomerular lesion. Histology is relatively non-specific in most cases, showing only damage and fibrosis in the interstitium apart from a few specific conditions.

Management

The most important aspect is the removal of the offending agent which may bring about improvement in renal function.

Corticosteroids These are often used especially if eosinophils and other inflammatory cells are seen on the renal biopsy, but controlled evidence for their use is lacking.

Prognosis

This is variable partly depending on the causative agent:

- Cases with acute onset and an identifiable causative drug have the best prognosis
- A long history of analgesic abuse or herbal remedy ingestion has a much worse prognosis

Some patients may temporarily or permanently need dialysis and those who recover often do not return to their previous baseline renal function. Analgesic and Chinese herbal nephropathy is associated with the development of renal and urothelial cancer.

10.3 Reflux nephropathy

The reflux of urine into the kidneys in childhood can cause lasting damage and produce significant impairment of function and renal failure in adult life.

Epidemiology

Reflux nephropathy accounts for about 5% of renal failure in the adult population on dialysis. The genetics are not well understood but the condition has quite a strong familial tendency. For this reason, adults with a family history of reflux nephropathy should be advised to have their children tested in the early postpartum period.

Causes and pathogenesis

The degree of reflux is graded by reference to an international agreed standard. It is thought that the compound papillae at the renal poles are vulnerable to back pressure effects due to closing inefficiently when urine refluxes up the ureters from the bladder. This in turn leads to scarring mainly at the upper and lower poles of the kidneys. It is thought that in the most part the damage is done by the age of four years.

Clinical features

The age of presentation of reflux nephropathy varies from early childhood to middle age. Children present either with a urinary tract infection or as part of investigations for enuresis. Adults present with the symptoms of renal impairment or disturbances of micturition or following routine tests, but there is usually a history of childhood urinary problems.

Investigations

Micturating cystogram In young children the gold standard investigation is the micturating cystogram; this not only secures the diagnosis but grades the degree of reflux. In older children and adults a dimercaptosuccinic acid (DMSA) scan is the best investigation for establishing the diagnosis, but cannot diagnose whether the patient is still refluxing. Dynamic renal scanning (triamine pentaacetic acid (DTPA) or technetium-99m mercaptoacetyltriglycine (MAG3)) with a reflux protocol can often demonstrate ongoing reflux but these radionuclides are less good for demonstrating scars.

Management and prognosis

The previous vogue for antireflux surgery has been superseded by a management strategy focused on keeping children free from infection with prophylactic antibiotics. Surgery is still offered to children with a high degree of reflux and those who fail medical therapy.

Prognosis in adults is governed by the initial creatinine at presentation, degree of proteinuria, blood pressure control and smoking; it is worse in male patients. Management in adults is therefore focused on good blood pressure control preferably with an angiotensin-converting enzyme (ACE) inhibitor.

10.4 Papillary necrosis

Papillary necrosis is characterised by the sloughing of the medullary papilla in to the renal pelvis which may cause haematuria and the same symptoms as calculus or clot.

Epidemiology
This is an uncommon renal condition, but one that must be considered in particular at-risk groups.

Causes and pathogenesis
Sickle cell disease patients are particularly prone to papillary necrosis. Often on the background of a pre-existing urine concentrating defect, an episode of hypotension or infection results in the sloughing of a papilla. Patients with diabetes and pyelonephritis are also vulnerable, as are patients who have consumed excessive compound analgesics.

Clinical features
Presentation is often with isolated haematuria or symptoms of loin pain identical to that from a calculus and/or infection.

Investigations

Intravenous urogram Classical imaging with an intravenous urogram (IVU) shows a non-calcified filling defect in the renal pelvis. On ultrasound an obstructed system may be noted. These patients will often need insertion of a nephrostomy for management of the hydronephrosis created by the obstructing papilla; the subsequent nephrostogram should demonstrate the sloughed papilla.

Management and prognosis

Patients with papillary necrosis require combined management between nephrological, urological and radiological colleagues. The sloughed papilla is sometimes passed and available for histology, but often it is presumed to disintegrate during the instrumentation required to remove it. Any underlying infection needs to be fully treated, and in people with diabetes, glycaemic control should be carefully examined. It is crucial to remember that these patients will have a predisposition to volume depletion in the future as they may fail to concentrate urine properly.

10.5 Infection

Numerically, infections of the renal tract are common, mostly of the lower urinary tract, particularly in women of childbearing years and are often due to Enterobacteriaceae. These are mostly easily treated in primary care; however, some patients also attend the secondary care setting as described below.

Recurrent urinary tract infections
Epidemiology

These are almost exclusively diagnosed in healthy young women who have experienced two or more urinary tract infections (UTIs) in six months or three or more in one year.

Causes and pathogenesis

A first infection with *Escherichia coli* seems to predispose to further infections. However, the frequency of sexual intercourse is the greatest risk factor for further episodes; other risk factors are a maternal history of UTIs, first infection before the age of 15, a new sexual partner in the last year and use of spermicides for contraception.

Clinical features

Urinary frequency, urgency and dysuria often accompanied by suprapubic pain are characteristic symptoms of UTI; loin pain or fever suggest pyelonephritis.

Investigations

Microbiological tests of the urine are diagnostic. Tests other than microbiology have a low yield; however, if there are unusual features such as an older age at presentation, haematuria between episodes, family history of stone disease or disabling infections, further urological tests should be undertaken. These are focused on looking for renal tract abnormalities or calculi on imaging (either an ultrasound or computed tomography (CT)) or by performing a cystoscopy.

Management

Micturition post-intercourse and adequate fluid intake are the most commonly recommended conservative treatments, but neither have a controlled evidence base. Likewise, cranberry juice is often advocated without controlled evidence. If associated with spermicides a different mechanism of contraception can be tried, while in postmenopausal women association with vaginal dryness may be alleviated with topical oestrogens.

If the infections are frequent despite the above measures then one of two strategies can be tried:

- A stand-by course of antibiotics is prescribed which can be taken immediately on suspicion of a UTI and following a midstream urine (MSU) sample that is dropped off to the laboratory. Failure to resolve the infection rapidly prompts elicitation of antibiotic sensitivities from the sample
- A regular rotating night-time antibiotic may be prescribed for when the urine is in the bladder for the longest time between micturition when bacteria have the longest time to multiply. Suitable drugs would include a penicillin, cephalosporin, trimethoprim and ciprofloxacin

Pyelonephritis

Pyelonephritis is when the substance of the medulla and cortex is infected. This is almost always caused by ascending bacteria and responds to systemic antibiotics, however, it can be very severe and lead to lasting complications in certain groups of patients.

Epidemiology

At the extremes of life it is more common in males, but otherwise it is more common in females.

Causes and pathogenesis

Pyelonephritis is more common when there is a functional or anatomical abnormality. These include urethral valves, reflux or prostatic enlargement in males and recurrent cystitis and reflux in females.

Clinical features

Presentation is usually with loin pain and fever which may be preceded by symptoms of a lower urinary tract infection.

Investigations

Urine should be sent for culture, and if admitted to hospital, the patient should have standard blood tests including creatinine, C-reactive protein (CRP), full blood count and blood cultures. Further investigations are undertaken as indicated by the history, the most common being an ultrasound followed by a CT urogram if there is a history of stone disease.

Management and prognosis

Most cases of pyelonephritis respond well to antibiotics and fluids. Patients ill enough to be admitted to hospital should be given intravenous antibiotics and fluids. A rapid response is expected and failure to respond suggests incorrect antibiotic choice or an infected obstructed system; the latter is a urological/radiological emergency.

The initial management of an infected obstructed system is the radiological placement of a nephrostomy drain and then investigation and treatment of the cause of the urinary flow impediment.

10.6 Renal tuberculosis

Classically renal tuberculosis is seen as a late reactivation of an old primary infection.

Epidemiology

This condition is seen mostly in areas with a high endemic rate of tuberculosis or in migrants from those areas in later life.

Pathogenesis

Renal involvement is never the primary infection, but results from haematological spread from another source; it can, however, spread onwards to the lower urinary tract, and in men to the epididymis.

Clinical features

Presentation is either with a classical sterile pyuria associated with dysuria and frequency or with weight loss and fever. Sterile pyuria with the presence of polymorphonuclear leucocytes has other causes besides tuberculosis: common false positives such as the sample being take while the patient is on antibiotics, chlamydia or cystitis must first be excluded.

Investigations

Urinalysis It is important that the laboratory is aware that the urine sample requires prolonged culture; some laboratories require the sample to be the first passed urine of the day. Three or four samples are required to ensure a reasonable diagnostic yield.

Imaging It is important to exclude tuberculosis-related strictures. Increasingly this is done by ultrasound and MAG3 radionuclide scanning rather than intravenous pyelography.

Management and prognosis

Standard antituberculosis therapy is required as indicated by local guidelines; this often includes pyrazinamide. Pyrazinamide is notable for blocking the tubular secretion of uric acid, although urate nephropathy is not of particular concern as urate is retained in the blood rather than appearing in the urine. By this mechanism the pyrazinamide may precipitate gout. Ureteric stricturing may occur for the first time after the start of antitubercular chemotherapy, and steroid therapy may be helpful for reducing the risk of stricture in these patients.

10.7 Renal sarcoidosis

Renal sarcoidosis is a granulomatous disease of unknown aetiology that is more common in particular ethnic groups. In this respect it overlaps with tuberculosis in Afro-Caribbean populations. It can affect any part of the renal tract and cause morbidity by causing interstitial disease or, rarely, obstructive uropathy.

Pathogenesis

The macrophages of the granulomas in sarcoidosis are capable of hydroxylating vitamin D into calcitriol and thereby inducing hypercalcaemia. This in turn can lead to nephrocalcinosis and nephrolithiasis. Notably these granulomas may be extrarenal although screening studies suggest renal involvement is more common than clinically suspected.

Clinical features

Renal involvement usually occurs as part of the multisystem nature of sarcoidosis or as a result of the hypercalcaemic nephropathy associated with the disease. Renal impairment is usually modest and only rarely does sarcoidosis lead to end-stage renal failure.

Investigations

On renal histology the granulomas of sarcoidosis can look very like the granulomas of tuberculosis but do not show caseation or bacteria on Ziehl–Nielson staining.

Management

The primary management of sarcoidosis is by glucocorticoid treatment, initially in doses of up to 1 mg/kg/day of prednisolone. Weaning the steroid dose can be difficult and some patients may need long-term treatment with a low dose. Multi-system involvement also guides the dose of steroids needed.

Hereditary disease

Inherited renal disease accounts for approximately 10% of cases of end-stage renal failure and causes biochemical abnormalities in individuals with less severe renal disease. Genetic mutations affect all components of the kidney. The commonest inherited renal disease is autosomal dominant (adult) polycystic kidney disease (ADPKD) where multiple cysts develop in the kidney and gradually damage functional renal tissue, leading to renal failure. There is also an autosomal recessive type of polycystic kidney disease (ARPKD) that presents in childhood.

Defects in the glomerular filter occur in the basement membrane, causing Alport syndrome and thin basement membrane disease. Defects in the podocyte occur in congenital focal segmental glomerulosclerosis.

There are a number of inherited defects of the ion channels and transporters in the renal tubule. The kidney is also involved in syndromes with defective tumour suppressor genes, the commonest being von Hippel–Lindau disease.

11.1 Clinical scenario

Raised blood pressure and haematuria

Presentation

A 45-year-old man is found to have a blood pressure of 164/88 mmHg with a urine dipstick test positive for haematuria but showing no proteinuria at a life-insurance medical examination.

Diagnostic approach

The key aspects to consider are secondary causes of hypertension, which include renal disease, and to diagnose the origin of the haematuria.

Further history

There is no family history of renal disease, stroke or unexplained sudden death. There has been one episode of macroscopic haematuria associated with right loin pain for 24 hours that had resolved spontaneously three months previously.

Examination
On examination the lower pole of the right kidney is bimanually palpable.

Diagnostic approach
The differential diagnosis of a palpable renal mass with haematuria includes renal carcinoma and autosomal dominant polycystic kidney disease (ADPKD). The episode of macroscopic haematuria with loin pain is compatible with an episode of bleeding into a renal cyst.

Investigations
Normal (i.e. non-dysmorphic) erythrocytes are found on urine microscopy. Serum creatinine is mildly elevated at 128 μmol/L. An abdominal ultrasound scan shows bilateral renal enlargement with multiple cysts of variable size. Cysts are also present in the liver.

Diagnostic approach
The ultrasound findings here are diagnostic of ADPKD.

11.2 Polycystic kidney disease

In PKD, multiple cysts develop in the renal tubule or collecting duct, which gradually increase in size due to active transport of water into the cysts. These cysts compress neighbouring renal tissue, eventually leading to renal failure. Autosomal recessive PKD (ARPKD) presents in childhood while the autosomal dominant form (ADPKD) presents later, usually in adult life, and often after individuals have had children.

In ADPKD, multiple cysts develop in the kidneys, liver, pancreas and seminal vesicle that gradually increase in size over time. Kidneys from a patient with ADPKD are shown in **Figure 11.1**. In ARPKD, multiple renal cysts arise from the collecting ducts. An associated feature is hepatic fibrosis due to biliary tract malformation.

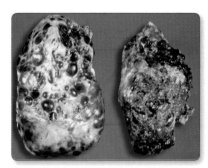

Figure 11.1 Kidneys removed from a patient with autosomal dominant polycystic kidney disease (ADPKD).

Autosomal dominant polycystic kidney disease

Epidemiology

ADPKD occurs in between 1 in 400 and 1000 live births, but may be diagnosed during life in only 50% of cases.

Pathogenesis

PKD is a ciliopathy due to defects in genes involved in controlling cilia. In ADPKD, 85% of affected individuals have a mutation in the PKD1

> **Clinical insight**
>
> ADPKD is the commonest inherited renal disease and accounts for 5–10% cases of end-stage renal failure.

locus on chromosome 16 which encodes polycystin-1, and the remaining patients have a mutation in the PKD2 locus on chromosome 4 which encodes polycystin-2. Cysts develop later and tend to progress more slowly with PKD2. While the genetic defect is present in all cells (i.e. it is a systemic disease), fewer than 10% of tubules are affected, leading to the hypothesis that a 'second hit' is required to drive cyst formation. Renal failure results from the cysts compressing and damaging normal renal tissue.

Clinical features

The kidneys and liver may be palpable. Up to 20% of patients have cerebral aneurysms with potential for rupture causing subarachnoid haemorrhage. A family history of intracranial aneurysms or stroke increases the likelihood of their presence.

Investigations

The diagnosis of ADPKD is usually made based on imaging findings. Ultrasound is the most straightforward approach, though smaller cysts can be detected with computed tomography (CT) or magnetic resonance imaging (MRI). Genetic linkage analysis can be undertaken where there is an informative pedigree. The genes can be sequenced in an individual without a family history but the linkage of mutations to disease phenotype is not always certain.

Ultrasound scanning can be used to screen individuals at genetic risk. This is a complex issue and the benefits of earlier disease detection allowing closer monitoring of blood pressure and other complications of ADPKD should be balanced against the psychological impact of a positive diagnosis and practical problems such as difficulty in obtaining life insurance. Conventional practice would be to offer screening to individuals from the age of 18 years and rescreening every five years in the absence of cysts until the age of 30 years based on the diagnostic criteria outlined below.

Diagnostic criteria

A number of criteria have been proposed based on imaging, the best established being the Ravine criteria for ultrasound findings, with the following age-dependent cut-offs for number of cysts to make the diagnosis of ADPKD in individuals at genetic risk:

- Less than 30 years of age: at least two cysts in one kidney or one cyst in each kidney
- 30–59 years of age: at least two cysts in each kidney
- 60 years or older: at least four cysts in each kidney

In individuals aged at least 40 years, the presence of one or no cysts excludes the disease. At ages 30–39, absence of cysts excludes the disease and in those younger than 30 years the disease cannot be excluded by ultrasound scanning.

Management

The mainstays of management aimed at slowing the progression of renal disease are:

- Treating blood pressure to <130/80 mmHg
- Early treatment of urinary tract infections

Vasopressin antagonists or physiological suppression of vasopressin by a high water intake may retard cyst growth and are the subject of ongoing clinical trials. Mammalian target of rapamycin (mTOR) inhibitors retard cyst growth, particularly in the liver, but do not preserve renal function.

Nephrectomy may be indicated for persistent pain, bleeding or urinary sepsis. Enlargement of the kidneys may compress the gut, causing problems with eating or leaving insufficient space for a renal transplant necessitating nephrectomy.

> ### Clinical insight
>
> Polycystic nephrectomy is a technically challenging operation associated with substantial morbidity and mortality. If possible it should be avoided.

Prognosis and complications

End-stage renal failure requiring dialysis typically develops after the age of 40 years in people with ADPKD. Risk of malignancy is greater than that for normal kidneys. The presence of multiple complex renal cysts can render identification of renal cell carcinomas by imaging difficult.

Autosomal recessive polycystic kidney disease
Epidemiology
ARPKD occurs in 1:10,000–1:40,000 live births.

Pathogenesis
ARPKD is caused by mutations in the PKHD1 gene located on chromosome 6 that encodes fibrocystin. In contrast to ADPKD, microcysts <3 mm in diameter develop. Hepatic fibrosis results from malformations of the developing biliary system.

Clinical features
ARPKD is diagnosed in a third of patients each:
- At age less than one year
- Between the ages of one and 20 years
- After the age of 20 years

Antenatal ultrasound detects most cases. Children presenting early are more likely to develop renal failure and later presenters are more likely to have hepatic complications. Hepatomegaly and portal hypertension develop in most patients. Renal manifestations are initially due to tubular dysfunction with hyponatraemia due to defective sodium reabsorption and reduced urine concentrating ability. Failure to secrete hydrogen ions leads to metabolic acidosis. Other manifestations of tubular dysfunction are mild proteinuria, glycosuria, phosphaturia and failure to retain magnesium. Hypertension occurs in two thirds of cases. Pulmonary hypoplasia is a major source of morbidity and mortality.

Investigations
Ultrasound scanning demonstrates large echogenic kidneys containing multiple small cysts. Hepatic fibrosis is seen as patches of high echogenicity in the liver. In older children, cysts may increase in size and be confused with ADPKD. MRI and CT scanning are also diagnostic.

Genetic testing including genetic mutation analysis and linkage analysis has variable detection rates.

Management
There is no established treatment to delay disease progression.

Prognosis and complications
Children surviving the first month have an 80% chance of surviving to age 15 years. Urinary tract infections are common and bacterial cholangitis can complicate biliary disease. Renal survival at 5, 10 and 20 years is 86%, 71% and 42%, respectively.

11.3 Inherited glomerular disease

Alport syndrome
Alport syndrome is hereditary nephritis with sensorineural deafness and ocular abnormalities due to inherited defects in type IV collagen, a key structural protein of the extra-cellular matrix that supports epithelial membranes.

Epidemiology

The frequency of abnormal genes is 1:5,000–1:10,000, with a disease prevalence of 1:10,000–1:50,000.

Pathogenesis

There are three patterns of inheritance, depending on which type IV collagen genes are involved:
- X-linked mutations of COL4A5 (80% of cases)
- Autosomal recessive mutations of COL4A3 or COL4A4 (15%)
- Autosomal dominant mutations in the COL4A3 or COL4A4 genes (5%)

These collagen abnormalities result in defective basement membranes.

Clinical features

Haematuria may be invisible or visible with progressive renal impairment. Hearing loss starts with high frequencies but progresses to lower frequencies. An anterior conal bulging of the lens (lenticonus) is the commonest ocular abnormality but the cornea and retina can also be involved.

Investigations

Diagnosis is usually confirmed by renal biopsy, with skin biopsy to identify collagen abnormalities as a less invasive alternative. Genetic mutation analysis can also be performed.

Management

No treatments have been clearly shown to modify disease progression to end-stage renal failure.

Prognosis and complications

End-stage renal failure usually develops between the ages of 16 and 35 years. A rare potential complication of renal transplantation is the development of antibodies to the glomerular basement membrane due to the absence of immunological tolerance to normal collagen in the donor kidney.

Thin basement membrane disease

Thin basement membrane disease is also known as benign familial haematuria.

Epidemiology

Less than 1% of the population are known to be affected, but the incidence may be as high as 5–9% based on data from live kidney donors.

Pathogenesis

Mutations in the type IV collagen genes COL4A3 and COL4A4 have been identified in some, but not all, families. Inheritance is autosomal dominant. In effect, these patients are heterozygous carriers of autosomal recessive Alport syndrome.

Clinical features

A family history of haematuria is present in 30–50% of cases. There is persistent or intermittent invisible haematuria. Visible haematuria is rare. If it does occur it may be associated with loin pain and in some cases is the underlying cause of loin pain–haematuria syndrome.

Investigations

Dysmorphic erythrocytes and erythrocyte casts may be noted on urine microscopy. Renal biopsy is not indicated for isolated invisible haematuria unless live donation for renal transplantation is planned. Biopsy is indicated in the presence of significant proteinuria. Diffuse thinning of the glomerular basement membrane to 150–225 nm (normal 300–400 nm) is found on electron microscopy examination of the renal biopsy, which is otherwise normal.

Management

No treatment is required. Annual checks of renal function, urinary protein and blood pressure are prudent.

Prognosis and complications

The prognosis is excellent and patients developing renal

complications usually have an alternative renal diagnosis such as Alport syndrome or IgA nephropathy.

Congenital focal segmental glomerulosclerosis (congenital nephrotic syndrome)

Congenital nephrotic syndrome is an autosomal recessive trait due to inherited defects in proteins involved in the glomerular filter.

Epidemiology

It occurs in fewer than 1 in 10,000 live births.

Pathogenesis

Ninety-five per cent of cases are due to mutations in NPHS1 or NPHS2:

- Mutations in the NPHS1 gene that codes for nephrin expressed in podocytes cause Finnish-type congenital nephrotic syndrome
- Mutations in the NPHS2 gene encoding podocin that interacts with nephrin in the slit diaphragm, also cause congenital nephrotic syndrome
- Mutations in the WT1 gene which encodes a tumour suppressor cause Denys–Drash syndrome, a triad of nephropathy, male pseudohermaphroditism and Wilms tumour
- Mutations in the gene encoding laminin beta 2, LAMB2, cause Pierson syndrome, where nephropathy is associated with ocular malformations

Clinical features

Most infants with congenital nephrotic syndrome are born prematurely and are small for their gestational age. Oedema is present at birth or within the first week of life in 50% of cases, and patients are always nephrotic within three months. Urinary protein loss including immunoglobulins leads to malnutrition and susceptibility to infection. Thromboembolism, and hypothyroidism due to loss of protein-bound thyroxine are potential complications.

Investigations

Renal ultrasound shows large echogenic kidneys with loss of normal corticomedullary differentiation. Renal biopsy taken early in the course of the disease shows mild mesangial changes with progressive glomerulosclerosis later.

Management

Congenital nephrotic syndrome is resistant to treatment with steroids or immunosuppressive drugs. Conservative measures to support development of the infant include albumin and immunoglobulin replacement, high protein, low-sodium diet and replacement of vitamins and thyroxine. Anticoagulation should be considered.

In some cases, bilateral nephrectomy is required to control nephrotic syndrome with initiation of renal replacement therapy. As an alternative, 'medical nephrectomy', using a combination of angiotensin-converting enzyme inhibition and the non-steroidal anti-inflammatory drug, indometacin, has been used to reduce the glomerular filtration rate sufficiently to reduce the protein leak.

> **Clinical insight**
>
> Congenital nephrotic syndrome is not inflammatory in nature so does not respond to treatment with steroids or immunosuppressive drugs.

Prognosis and complications

End-stage renal failure usually occurs between three and eight years of age. Recurrence after transplantation due to the development of antinephrin antibodies has been reported.

11.4 Inherited tubular disease

A number of inherited disorders result in defective tubular secretion or reabsorption.

Disordered tubular sodium transport

A defect in chloride-associated sodium transport in the loop of of Henle, mimicking loop diuretic treatment, is found in Bartter syndrome, and in the early distal tubule in Gitelman syndrome, which mimics thiazide diuretic treatment. Liddle syndrome results in increased sodium reabsorption in the collecting duct.

Epidemiology
The incidence of Gitelman syndrome is 1 in 40,000 and Bartter syndrome 1 in 1,000,000. Approximately 1% of the population are heterozygous carriers for these autosomal recessive conditions. The Liddle syndrome is rare.

Pathogenesis and clinical features

Bartter and Gitelman syndromes In these syndromes, volume contraction leads to secondary hyperaldosteronism, which further leads to hypokalaemia and metabolic alkalosis, but patients are normotensive. Urine concentrating capacity is impaired in Bartter syndrome with resulting water loss leading to polyuria and polydipsia. Urinary calcium excretion is normal or high with Bartter syndrome, which may result in secondary hyperparathyroidism, but is reduced in Gitelman syndrome and may cause hypercalcaemia. Hypomagnesaemia is a feature of both Gitelman and Bartter syndromes. Key differential diagnoses for Bartter and Gitelman syndromes are self-induced vomiting or diuretic use.

Liddle syndrome This involves increased reabsorption of sodium in the collecting duct due to an autosomal dominantly inherited gain-of-function mutation. This leads to apparent mineralocorticoid excess with hypertension and hypokalaemia but low plasma aldosterone concentration.

> ### Guiding principles
> Consider these syndromes in any patient with hypokalaemia. Remembering that Bartter syndrome mimics loop diuretic treatment and Gitelman syndrome mimics thiazide diuretic treatment is a useful aide memoir to the biochemical abnormalities in each syndrome.

Investigations
Urinary calcium excretion can differentiate between Bartter and Gitelman syndrome.

Management

Patients with Bartter syndrome have elevated renal prostaglandin E_2 concentration, which can be treated with non-steroidal anti-inflammatory drugs. This is not the case for Gitelman syndrome. Potassium-sparing diuretics such as amiloride or spironolactone treat the hypokalaemia, metabolic alkalosis and have some impact on hypomagnesaemia. Most patients require potassium and magnesium supplementation. Liddle syndrome is treated with triamterene or amiloride.

Cystinuria

Cystinuria is an inherited disorder of tubular reabsorption of the amino acid cystine, which results in formation of renal stones. It is present in 1 in 7,000 births.

Pathogenesis

The cystine transporter also transports the other dibasic amino acids, but ornithine, arginine and lysine are more soluble than cystine and do not usually crystallise to form stones. Inheritance, in terms of propensity to form stones, is autosomal recessive. Most affected individuals have homozygous mutations in the SLC3A1 or SLC7A9 genes, which encode two chains of the amino acid transporter. Heterozygotes have raised (but soluble) urinary cystine concentrations.

Investigations

Hexagonal crystals may be seen on urine microscopy. Stone analysis demonstrates the presence of cystine. Urine cystine concentration is usually >1.7 mmol/day (normal <0.13 mmol/day).

Management

The mainstay of treatment is generation of dilute urine, lowering cystine concentration to below the point where crystals start to form. Measurement of 24-hour cystine excretion can be used to calculate the daily urine output to keep urinary cystine concentration <1 mmol/L and in solution. Patients need to be advised to drink overnight as well as during the day to avoid high nocturnal urinary cystine concentration.

Dietary sodium and protein restriction reduces cystine excretion but influence on stone formation is uncertain. Cystine is more soluble in alkaline urine, which can be achieved by administration of potassium citrate or potassium bicarbonate.

In the event of these conservative measures failing to control urine cystine concentration, D-penicillamine can be used to increase the solubility of cystine.

Prognosis and complications

The complications are those of renal stones (see Chapter 12), rarely leading to end-stage renal failure.

> ## Clinical insight
>
> Renal stones are due to crystallisation of substances present at supersaturated concentrations in urine. Increasing water intake to generate dilute urine is the mainstay of prevention of stones in predisposed individuals.

11.5 Tumour syndromes

Tuberous sclerosis complex

Description

Tuberous sclerosis complex is an autosomal dominant condition causing angiomyolipomas, benign tumours containing vascular, smooth muscle and adipose components in the kidney. Other benign tumours (hamartomas) occur in the brain and a number of other tissues.

Epidemiology

Tuberous sclerosis complex affects 1 in 5,000 to 1 in 10,000 live births.

Pathogenesis

Mutations are present in either the TSC1 or TSC2 genes. A positive family history is present in fewer than 40% of cases. The TSC genes function as tumour suppressers, through inhibition of mTOR.

Clinical features

Benign hamartomas are found in a number of organs including the brain, eyes, heart, kidney, liver, lung and skin. Angiomyolipomas of the kidney are present in 60–80% of cases and may present with pain, renal bleeding or renin-driven hypertension. There is an increased risk of malignancy with renal cell carcinoma in 1–2% of affected adults.

Epilepsy is common and at least 50% have some degree of cognitive impairment or learning disability. The classical neurological lesion is periventricular glioneuronal hamartomas, known as tubers. Giant cell astrocytomas and diffuse abnormalities of cerebral white matter may also develop. Autistic spectrum disorders are common in children.

Skin lesions are common, classically: angiofibromas on the face or under nails, hypopigmented macules (ash leaf spots), shagreen patches on the trunk or a brown plaque on the forehead. Some adults develop pulmonary lymphangioleiomyomatosis.

Investigations
Renal ultrasound or CT scanning demonstrate angiomyolipomas. Cranial MRI and electroencephalogram are used to investigate neurological involvement.

Diagnostic criteria
Standard diagnostic criteria for tuberous sclerosis complex are shown in **Table 11.1**.

Management
Large angiomyolipomas that are at risk of bleeding or have bled can be treated by blocking their blood supply (embolisation) using an interventional radiology approach. Angiomyolipomas or renal cell carcinomas may require surgical resection. Nephron-sparing partial nephrectomy, usually with a laparoscopic approach, is the preferred option due to the potential to develop further problems in the contralateral kidney. Recent clinical trial data have shown reduction in growth of angiomyolipomas using the mTOR inhibitor, everolimus.

Prognosis and complications
Progressive enlargement of angiomyolipomas, which can be associated with haemorrhage, may lead to loss of renal function.

Major features	Minor features
Facial angiofibromas or forehead plaque	Multiple, randomly distributed pits in dental enamel
Non-traumatic ungual or periungual fibroma	Hamartomatous rectal polyps
Hypomelanotic macules (three or more)	Bone cysts
Shagreen patch (connective tissue nevus)	Cerebral white matter radial migration lines
Multiple retinal nodular hamartomas	Gingival fibromas
Glioneuronal hamartoma (cortical tuber)	Non-renal hamartoma
Subependymal nodule	Retinal achromic patch
Subependymal giant cell astrocytoma	'Confetti' skin lesions
Cardiac rhabdomyoma, single or multiple	Multiple renal cysts
Lymphangiomyomatosis	
Renal angiomyolipoma	

Table 11.1 Major and minor clinical features of tuberous sclerosis complex. Definite tuberous sclerosis complex: two major or one major plus two minor features. Probable tuberous sclerosis complex: one major plus one minor feature. Possible tuberous sclerosis complex: either one major feature or two or more minor features.

von Hippel–Lindau disease

von Hippel–Lindau (VHL) disease is an autosomal dominant syndrome leading to a variety of benign and malignant neoplasms including:

- Haemangioblastoma in the central nervous system
- Renal cell carcinoma
- Phaeochromocytoma
- Endolymphatic sac tumours of the middle ear
- Papillary cystadenomas of the epididymis and broad ligament
- Retinal angiomas

- Serous cystadenomas
- Neuroendocrine tumours of the pancreas

Epidemiology

This condition is present in 1 in 36,000 live births.

Pathogenesis

As with ADPKD a 'two-hit' hypothesis applies here. All cells have one abnormal copy of the von Hippel–Lindau tumour suppressor gene, requiring a 'second-hit' to the normal copy leading to oncogenesis.

Clinical features

Mean age at presentation is in the mid-twenties. Haemangioblastomas are the commonest disease manifestation, affecting 60–80% of individuals.

Investigations

MRI is recommended to screen for haemangioblastomas in the central nervous system.

Diagnostic criteria

VHL is divided into two types according to the risk of developing phaeochromocytoma; patients with type I disease have a low incidence, whereas it is common in those with type II disease. Type II disease is further divided based on the risk of renal cell carcinoma; IIA is low risk, IIB patients have a high risk. Kindreds with type IIC disease have phaeochromocytomas only without renal cell carcinoma or haemangioblastomas.

Management

Annual retinal screening for development of angiomas is recommended to allow early treatment to preserve vision. Renal cell carcinoma develops in 60% of patients beyond the age of 60 years. Renal screening with CT or MRI is recommended to allow early nephron-sparing surgery. Annual imaging for phaeochromocytoma should commence in adolescence.

chapter 12

Urological nephrology

A simple definition of urology would be 'the study of diseases of the urogenital tract potentially requiring surgical intervention'. The specialty is divided into urodynamics, oncology, stone disease, reconstruction, paediatric urology and andrology. Urological conditions are relatively common and admissions account for up to a third of all surgical hospital admissions. Urologists work very closely with nephrologists because of the potential impact of urological conditions on renal function. Although very few urological conditions are immediately life-threatening on presentation, they can severely affect the quality of life of those affected, making their early diagnosis and management essential.

12.1 Clinical scenario

Left loin pain

Presentation

A 44-year-old male accountant presents with severe colicky left loin pain that is radiating into his groin.

Examination

There is no focal abdominal tenderness, however the patient intermittently winces and bends over gripping his flank and groin. Apart from signs of dehydration, his examination is normal.

Further history

The patient had experienced a similar pain two years ago, but it had been short lived and seemed to resolve after he passed some gritty urine, so he had ignored it. He also mentions that he has recently been sitting at his desk working for long hours without eating or drinking, apart from a couple of pints of milk daily.

Diagnostic approach

It is likely he has ureteric stones (or calculi). Sudden-onset abdominal pain should be taken seriously; the nature of the pain in terms of its character and radiation can give clues to the cause. In this instance the pain is colicky or spasmodic in nature, with a classical radiation pattern. For example, it is not uncommon for men to describe radiation of pain to the tip of the penis.

It is important to exclude hypercalcaemia, for example in association with hyperparathyroidism or malignancy. Patients should be assessed for gout as evidence of hyperuricaemia. A dietary and sedentary lifestyle history as well as personal or family history of renal stones should be enquired about. It is also essential to exclude a history of recurrent urinary tract infections.

Investigations

A urine sample is sent for urinalysis to assess for the presence of crystals or infection. Computed tomography of the kidney, ureter and bladder (CT KUB) is performed to assess the size, number and precise location of the stone(s).

Management

The patient is confirmed to have a single calcium stone in his ureter, seen on CT KUB imaging. Extracorporeal shock wave lithotripsy is successful and he is discharged two days later with information on how to prevent future stone formation.

12.2 Stone disease (calculi)

Renal calculi have been found in early Egyptian mummies from as far back as 5000 BC. The management, and particularly the prevention, of this condition is largely based on our understanding of the metabolic pathways that predispose to it.

Epidemiology

Renal stone disease is most common in men and in the third to fifth decade of life. The incidence is higher among the affluent, with an overall prevalence of between 5% and 10% in most populations.

Causes

Factors that predispose to stone formation include:

- Dehydration
- Sedentary lifestyle
- High dietary calcium
- Oxalate or urate intake

Clinical insight

Diet and stones

Northern Europeans and those living in the Western world may be more prone to renal calculi because of their relatively high intake of animal proteins.

Pathogenesis

The development of renal stones is multifactorial. About 75% of stones are formed mainly of calcium while others consist of uric acid, cystine or struvite. It is not uncommon for stones to be formed of a mixture of different crystals.

Stone formation Stone formation is caused by the abundance of a solute, and is often exacerbated by dehydration. The initial phase is supersaturation, which is followed by subsequent crystallisation. Larger stones may develop as a result of one crystal type growing on top of another, a phenomenon known as 'epitaxy'. Interestingly, these mechanisms seem to contribute more to non-calcium-based stone formation.

Inhibitors In some instances, an individual may lack a 'stone inhibitor' such as citrate, pyrophosphate, magnesium, zinc, nephrocalcin, Tamm–Horsfall glycoprotein, uropentin and macromolecules, which are believed to prevent crystallisation.

Matrix initiation Another potential factor is non-crystalline mucoprotein (matrix), which may act as an initiator in some stone formers by providing a framework for crystal deposition, especially in association with *Proteus* bacterial infections. Renal tubular dysfunction, for instance in Fanconi's syndrome, leads to impaired secretion and absorption of some of the excreted substances.

Exogenous substances

An additional predisposing factor could be ingestion of exogenous substances such as protease inhibitors, e.g. indinavir, a drug used for treating HIV infection.

Clinical features

The most common presentation is with pain, usually colicky and in the loin. There may be radiation into the groin region, and in men to the testicles or tip of the penis. This is due to a combination of the stone moving and the nerve supply to the urogenital tract (see page 6).

A full history on the character of the pain is essential. Stones can occur anywhere along the urinary tract and the description of the pain can give clues as to the location:

- Kidney stones cause loin pain
- Ureteric stones cause renal colic
- Bladder stones tend to cause strangury; a slow and painful urination

Patients sometimes develop haematuria as a result of stone trauma on the endothelial lining of the urinary tract. Renal calculi may also be associated with infection which may have preceded or developed in the presence of the stone (see pathogenesis above). Patients may also present with vomiting or fever, even in the absence of infection.

Clinical insight

Pain radiation and renal calculi

The pattern of radiation of pain with renal calculi is due to the close embryological development of the urogenital and gastroenterology systems.

Investigations

Two separate 24-hour urine collections should be sent for urinalysis, to quantify the amount of calcium, oxalate, urate and/or cysteine in the urine. Urine should also be sent for microscopy, culture and sensitivity as there is often an associated urinary tract infection. Where patients have actually voided stones, these should be sent for biochemical analysis and/or X-ray crystallography.

Imaging involves plain KUB radiographs, intravenous urography, abdominal ultrasound of the urinary tract and axial or spiral CT scans (**Figure 12.1**).

Management

Adequate pain relief and antiemetics, where necessary, are important. Patients often require potent analgesics, such as

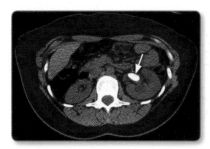

Figure 12.1 Computed tomography (CT) scan demonstrating a renal calculus (arrow) in the left kidney..

opiates. Good hydration is also important as this alone can help expel the stone(s). The threshold for starting antibiotics should be low, particularly where surgical or radiological intervention is planned.

Patients often need general resuscitation with pain relief, antiemetics and hydration. The actual treatment of the stones can be approached in five different ways depending on the size, location, degree of obstruction and the type of stone.

Conservative management This is often used for stones that are ≤5 mm. It entails hydration to flush the stone out and radiological monitoring to confirm passage of the stone. Most stones pass spontaneously.

Lithotripsy Extracorporeal shockwave lithotripsy is used for stones ≥2 cm in size. Repeated sessions may be needed, and there is a risk of stone fragments obstructing the ureter further down.

Retrograde renoscopy This is used for disintegrating stones of <1 cm in size. It involves the introduction of a laser fibre through an enteroscope into the bladder, ureter and renal collecting system.

Percutaneous nephrolithotomy This is used for stones >2 cm in size. It entails percutaneous transparenchymal (through the skin and kidney tissue) access to the collecting system by disintegrating devices and endoscopes using fluoroscopic guidance to remove usually superficial stones.

Surgery Open surgery is usually reserved for staghorn calculi, where the majority of the stones are located centrally in the calices and the kidney is contributing minimal function. Laparoscopic surgery is not usually possible due to extensive perinephric fibrosis.

Prognosis and complications

There is some risk of urinary sepsis.

The short-term outcome for patients is usually good as most are treatable. Patients who present late or have underlying metabolic disease are more problematic. In the long-term, recurrent stone formation is not uncommon, especially if preventive measures are not put into place.

Prevention Knowing the type of stone guides appropriate preventive measures. Although high fluid intake is the mainstay of prevention, the following drugs can also be used:
- Allopurinol for hyperuricaemia
- Penicillamine for cystinuria
- Thiazide diuretics for hypercalciuria

Lifestyle and dietary measures, including decreasing calcium and oxalate intake, increasing activity levels, and drinking more water can also be tried to reduce stone recurrence.

12.3 Tumours: urothelial neoplasia

Neoplasia can occur anywhere along the urogenital tract: the prostate (beyond the scope of this book), the bladder (**Figure 12.2**) and the kidney. Tumours of the renal pelvis, ureter and urethra are relatively rare. Various associations have been described including oestrogens, diet and obesity, renal failure (particularly for the kidneys), hereditary syndromes, smoking and toxic agents such as lead, cadmium, asbestos, cyclophosphamide and aniline dyes.

The presentation will depend on the size, location and stage of the tumour, a well as the baseline health of the patient. Common presentations include symptoms as a direct result of invasion of the urinary tract including pain, haematuria and obstructive symptoms as well as constitutional symptoms.

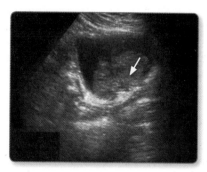

Figure 12.2 Ultrasound scan demonstrating bladder carcinoma (arrow).

Treatment may be curative or palliative involving surgery, radiotherapy, hormonal manipulation or chemotherapy. The prognosis is highly variable and depends on the same criteria as for management.

Renal neoplasia

This is an abnormal growth in either or both of the kidneys and may be benign or malignant. Up to 20% of kidney tumours may present with a paraneoplasia, a clinical or biochemical disturbance not directly as a result of invasion or metastasis of the primary tumour.

Epidemiology

It is essential to distinguish benign renal lesions, such as angiomyolipoma and cysts, from malignant lesions, as this determines subsequent management. Angiomyolipomas account for less than 0.5% of cases. Renal oncocytomas, a relatively benign neoplasm, form between 3% and 7% of renal tumours.

Renal carcinomas are the most common malignant renal tumours, with an incidence of approximately 3% of all tumours. Their incidence has increased significantly in the past 50 years.

Causes

There appears to be a strong association between renal carcinoma and tobacco use. In some instances, such as Von Hippel–Lindau disease (an autosomal dominant disease), a genetic association for carcinogenesis has been described.

Pathogenesis

The mutation or inactivation of two alleles of the 'tumour suppressor gene', known as 'the two hit theory', is believed to have a strong role in the pathogenesis of renal tumours.

Clinical features

The 'classic triad' of flank pain, haematuria and a palpable mass is now not often seen. Fortunately, most tumours are diagnosed before they become palpable, particularly in modern healthcare settings, and largely due to increased screening. A paraneoplastic presentation can, however, lead to challenges in diagnosis and sometimes the diagnosis is an incidental finding.

> **Clinical insight**
>
> A paraneoplastic syndrome is a clinical or biochemical manifestation leading to a disease or symptom as a consequence of primary or metastatic cancer cells in the body. The presentation can be an endocrine, neurological, mucocutaneous or haematological abnormality.

Approach to the patient

This requires a full history and examination along with an index of suspicion particularly in an older patient or those with a family history of cancer. Attention to detail is needed in a general physical examination, for instance, to assess for new-onset varicoceles in men, or signs of disease that could be consistent with paraneoplasia.

Investigations

A full blood count, erythrocyte sedimentation rate (ESR), serum calcium, liver function test and renal profiles should be carried out as baseline investigations.

Diagnosis is by imaging, although not every mass in the kidney is a tumour and sometimes a tissue diagnosis is required (**Table 12.1**). Ultrasound is usually the first-line investigation, but an abdominal CT scan is essential for staging (**Figure 12.3**). The CT may need to be extended if indicated by findings on

	Solid renal masses	Cystic renal masses
Benign lesions	Angiomyolipoma	Simple cyst
	Oncocytoma	Multilocular cystic neoplasm
	Xanthogranulomatous pyelonephritis	Calyceal diverticulum
	Benign mesenchymal tumours	
Malignant lesions	Renal adenocarcinoma	Cystadenocarcinomas
	Sarcoma	Cystic necrosis of renal carcinomas
	Metastatic lesions	Renal carcinoma in a simple cyst
	Lymphoma/leukaemia	

Table 12.1 Differential diagnosis of masses in the kidney.

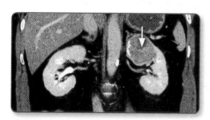

Figure 12.3 Computed tomography (CT) scan demonstrating a renal tumour (arrow) in the left kidney.

a chest X-ray. Magnetic resonance imaging (MRI) is useful for characterising venous involvement. CT and MRI are also critical for planning debulking or curative surgery.

Management

Conservative In some instances observation is the best approach, particularly where the rate of growth is slow and the there is minimal risk of metastasis. This applies to many of the tumours found incidentally in the older population, where their presence is unlikely to impact on lifespan, and the patient may be unfit for surgery.

Surgery Where feasible, removal of the tumour by open radical nephrectomy or partial nephrectomy offers the best chance of cure. A partial nephrectomy can mean renal function is preserved, but carries a higher risk of recurrence or incomplete resection of tumour. A debulking nephrectomy may be performed to reduce tumour load prior to immunotherapy.

Ablation Cryotherapy or radiofrequency ablation can be used to reduce tumour load, or may even be curative, but only if the tumour is in the periphery.

Adjuvant treatment Increasingly, adjuvant treatment with chemotherapy, immunotherapy (e.g. interferon alfa and interleukin 2) is used, especially for metastatic disease or for patients unfit to undergo surgery.

Clinical insight

Kidney metastasis

Metastasis to the kidneys should always be considered with lymphomas, melanomas, breast or lung cancer.

Prognosis and complications

Prognosis depends on the extent of the tumour at the time of diagnosis and the patient's fitness, which will determine the management strategy offered. Complications, such as systemic illness, wasting, infections, pain, and depression make supportive management essential.

12.4 Retroperitoneal fibrosis

This condition is also known as Ormond disease and involves proliferation of fibrous tissue in the retroperitoneum (region behind the posterior peritoneal cavity). It is sometimes described as periaortitis, but is often much more extensive, involving the compartment of the body containing the kidneys, aorta, renal tract and various other structures.

Epidemiology

Retroperitoneal fibrosis (RPF) is rare and twice as common in males as females. It is most commonly seen between the fifth and seventh decade of life.

Causes

About 30% of cases have a clear association, most commonly with aortic aneurysm, but also malignancy, infection, and medications such as methysergide, hydralazine, and β-blockers. Other causes include idiopathic retroperitoneal fibrosis, which probably has an autoimmune cause, and can be associated with diseases such as Riedel thyroiditis and sarcoidosis.

Pathogenesis

RPF is probably multifactorial in origin. Idiopathic retroperitoneal fibrosis, however, is an immune-mediated phenomenon. It is postulated that macrophages may be triggered to produce cytokines that stimulate proliferation of fibroblasts and the subsequent fibrosis that characterise this disease.

Clinical features

It may present with constitutional symptoms such as malaise and fever. Other symptoms include:
- Lower back pain, usually dull in nature and gradually increasing over time
- Renal failure
- Hypertension
- Pain
- Swelling and
- Change in colour of the legs

In some patients, deep vein thrombosis and other obstructive symptoms have also been described.

Investigations

The diagnosis of RPF should always prompt a search for the aetiology, as treatment of the underlying condition may be the only definitive means of controlling it.

Imaging CT is the investigation of choice to demonstrate the extent of fibrosis and its obstruction of the urinary tract (**Figure 12.4**). Kidney ultrasound is often part of preliminary screening for obstruction.

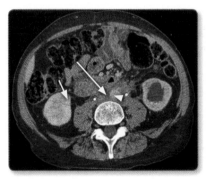

Figure 12.4 Computed tomography (CT) scan demonstrating retroperitoneal fibrosis. Retroperitoneal fibrotic tissue (arrow) and periaortitis (long arrow) around the aorta (arrowhead) are seen.

Biopsy This is indicated when malignancy or infection is suspected, or in cases refractory to treatment.

Blood tests Renal function should be assessed. Inflammatory markers such as C-reactive protein (CRP) and erythrocyte sedimentation rate (ESR) can be useful indicators of the degree of inflammation and response to treatment.

Management
The aims are to ensure no malignancy is involved, preserve renal function, prevent other organ involvement and relieve symptoms. Where possible, the underlying cause should be treated, for example:
- Identifying and withdrawing a drug causing RPF
- Surgical repair of an inflammatory aortic aneurysm

Corticosteroids are the first line of treatment for idiopathic retroperitoneal fibrosis. Disease modifying agents are often introduced later, either as steroid-sparing agents, or where the condition is refractory to corticosteroids; agents include include colchicine, azathioprine, mycophenolate mofetil, cyclophosphamide and tamoxifen. Fibrolysis with laser and even surgery are sometimes required to prevent complete obstruction of the urinary tract.

Prognosis and complications

The outcome depends on the extent of fibrosis and impact on the renal tract at the time of diagnosis. Delayed diagnosis often means irreversible damage with poor long-term outcomes.

Complications are usually related to obstructive damage of the urinary tract and can lead to varying degrees of renal failure.

Index

Note: Page numbers in **bold** or *italic* refer to tables or figures respectively.

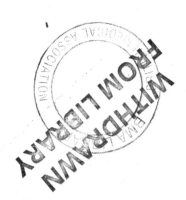